ABOUT THE AUTHOR

Robert was born in the early 1960's in East London.
He trained in Judo and boxing as a child and at age
18 began training in Yang Family Taijiquan.

For many years he studied the Chinese Internal Arts in depth.
In the 1990's he set up his own school and began cross
training in several styles.

In 2000 he began training in Systema and has since trained
extensively with with Mikhail Ryabko and Vladimir Vasiliev in both
Moscow and Toronto. In addition he has arranged numerous UK
seminars for Mikhail, Vladimir and other instructors.

Robert now trains solely in Systema and runs regular classes
in the UK and teaches seminars throughout the UK and Europe.
He has been featured in numerous martial arts books and magazines
as well as producing his own publications and training films.

Outside of training, Robert is a professional musician and currently
lives in rural Bedfordshire with his wife and a small menagerie.

"Rob Poyton has been training and teaching Systema since 2000.
He is a dedicated and talented instructor, knowledgeable on
all of the key components of Systema. Rob presents his teaching
in a clear and structured manner through his classes
and reading materials."
- Vladimir Vasiliev, October 2019.

*Dedicated to Daisy Cane
and Ada Poyton*

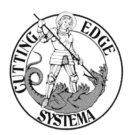

Published by Cutting Edge

ISBN:978-1-63752-606-4

CONTENTS

CHAPTER ONE
INTRODUCTION

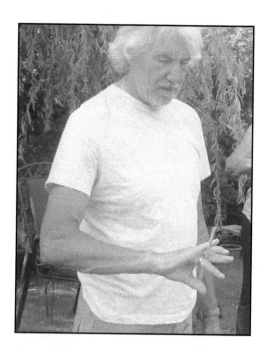

Systema is a Russian discipline that is fairly new to the west. Indeed, the first Systema class outside of Russia was only set up in the mid 1990's, by Vladimir Vasiliev in Toronto. Since then, thanks to his efforts and those of his teacher Mikhail Ryabko, Systema has spread around the world. To date, there are around 250 schools globally teaching Ryabko/Vasiliev Systema.

Systema came to most of us via a military background. Both main teachers have extensive service histories in Russian special forces units. It may come as some surprise, then, to learn that Systema has an extensive health and well-being aspect to its practice. This should not really be a surprise when we consider the roots of Systema.

In the west, most martial traditions became lost, separated from their origins, or retained only for ceremonial purposes. In Russia, many traditional arts where incorporated into modern military training, and this included health practices. After all, a warrior who is sick or ill is a warrior unable to defend the homeland! Furthermore, in recent years the art has been reconnected with its spiritual roots in the Russian Orthodox church, also the source of some of these health practices.

In fact, if you ask many Systema practitioners, they don't like calling what they do a martial art at all! Not because it lacks effectiveness - in my experience, it is the most comprehensive fighting art around - but because the practice of Systema goes way beyond any combat application, in a very direct way. Many martial arts pay lip-service to health, but then ask you to train in ways that damage the body. Others certainly contain meditative practices but these are generally divorced from the reality of movement and strife.

Systema offers a full package. Think of it more as an operating system than a style. You can use it to run whichever program you like, be that mobility, general health, self defence, sports, daily activities, professional work, recovering from illness and so on. The principles employed in Systema are simple, universal and profound. Above all, they are accessible to people of all ages and conditions. Even an immobile or bed-bound person can practice breathing exercises. Every training method can be easily adjusted to suit. Systema is something that adapts to you, not the other way round.

In addition, the main Systema teachers are not distant figures, lost in the haze of legend. They are here and now, very accessible, open to questions, and always developing. At age 57, I am younger (just!) than both my teachers, yet they continue to move in ways that defy the restrictions of conventional thought. For this is another issue. Time and time again I hear the phrase "well, you have to expect that at your age!" And this sometimes addressed to people in the thirties or forties! There is an assumption that as we age we should be less active, move less, do less, learn less, accept the back aches, stiffness and pain that "comes with age."

I'm here to tell you *no* to all that! Injury or ailment aside, there is nothing to say we should be less free in our movement at 85 than 5. Of course, if we have not moved in such a way for many years, there will be issues to overcome. And, of course, there are certain facts we have to face with an ageing body. But by and large, we can lead full, vigorous and active lives even into our nineties. If you don't believe me, run a search for the videos of the 90 year old gymnast, or the seniors in parks in China touching there toes and doing the splits! Exercise starts in the mind!

Conversely, as mentioned, people with

ailments or conditions are still able to get so much from Systema. The key is always to take thing step by step, to set ourselves minor goals that lead to big achievements. We will talk more on this later on.

WHO IS THIS BOOK FOR?

This book is aimed at two groups of people. One is people who have some familiarity with Systema. The other is people who are looking for a suitable and comprehensive training program and have little or no previous experience. To this end I apologise if some of the material is familiar to "Systema-ists" but even so, it never does any harm to re-visit the basics.

Actually, there is one other group who will also find this book useful - instructors who wish to teach seniors. They may be members of your family, it may be you are

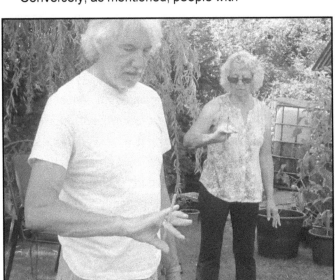

running a class in a care home or similar institution. I hope this will give you some guidance in formulating training for your family, friends and students.

Of course, there is nothing to say you have to be a certain age to use this book. All of the exercises here are suitable for young as well as old! However I will be gearing everything towards those

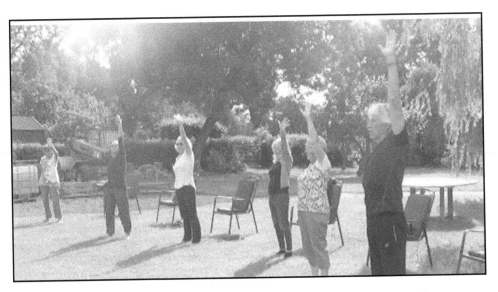

with perhaps a little less mobility, or who have not exercised for some time.

Given the current circumstances I am also concentrating on solo practice. Systema has numerous methods for working with one or more partners, but for the most part, I want to present you with activities that you can practice on your own, perhaps even in preparation for visiting a local class, or taking part in an on-line Zoom session.

While all of the work presented carries over into what we might call "self defence", in terms of dealing with an attacker, I will not be going into that aspect here. Having said that, I tend to approach "self defence" in its wider context. So learning to fall safely, for example, is just as much self defence in my view as learning to defend yourself with a stick.

HOW TO USE THIS BOOK?

I advise having a read through the whole book first off, then going back and trying some of the basic exercises. If you are already familiar with these, move on to the other exercises. If not, work with the basics until you are comfortable with the core exercises. Then begin exploring all the other aspects presented here.

Don't feel you have to do everything! There will no doubt be some areas of exercise you feel drawn to more than others, that's fine. The main thing is that you can keep your training interesting and engaging. If you find yourself getting a bit bored, then use some of the other methods here to tweak your sessions a little - that is one of the strengths of the Systema approach.

Just one note on the photos in this book. Normally, I like to take book photos during

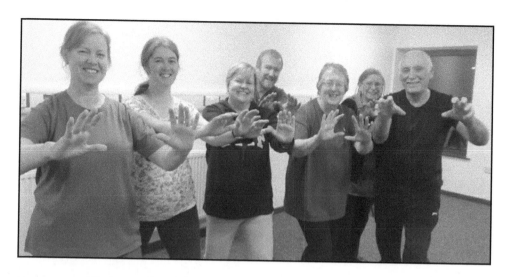

class for a more "live" feel. However this was written under lock down and so I've had to use either some photos from previous books or many more photos of myself than I would normally use! Hopefully they are clear enough to follow, that is the main thing.

EXERCISE vs ACTIVITY

I've been involved in physical training of one type or another since the age of around seven. In all that time, I've only ever attended a gym session a couple of times. To be honest "exercise" bores me rigid! Working to numbers, having a set routine that rarely varies, ticking boxes in a chart, it's not for me. So I try to avoid the "E word" where possible. I much prefer describing what we do as "activity."

Here's why. Exercise is something we set time aside for, it's a part of our routine. Get home from work, feed the cat, do thirty minutes cardio. Or, on a Tuesday morning spend 40 minutes lifting weights in the gym. That's okay but I find that this separates exercise out from our daily life. What I'm interested in is something that enhances all my daily activities, something that becomes part of me rather than something I do. That way, my training activity can't help but underpin my walking, general movement, running for the bus, going for a swim, taking the stairs two at a time, helping me recover from the flu, even having an impact on my personal relationships.

Because, simple as some of the work we do appears, it works deep. The breath work is a prime example. Even the most basic methods give you a powerful took to begin managing your day to day stress levels in a constructive way. Not by furiously hurling weights around as you listen to loud music, that tends to either mask stress or increase it. Instead, the activities detailed here will have an effect on each of the body/ mind systems in a way that is universally applicable, that helps bring us back to the default "operating system" we had as children. Kids run, laugh, climb, fall over,cry, roll around, swim, jump, explore, engage and react in a totally natural fashion, without excess tension and with seemingly boundless reserves of energy. That is the natural state we aim to return to.

THE BODY SYSTEMS

In one sense, we are a collection of systems. Nervous system, skeletal, cardio, digestive, muscular, glandular and so on. These are some of the body systems. Then we have our brain systems. Emotions, physiology, psychology, beliefs, cultural / social, ego, and so on. Systema (the name means "system") is the study of each of these - both individually and also how they inter-act with each other.

Once we have a grasp of our own systems, we also study how they interact with others, be that the environment or other people. In this way, the methods are virtually infinitely adjustable to suit our aims. A static breathing exercise calms the nervous system. Combine it with a

press up to also work the muscular system. In any activity, always try and be aware of your posture, tension and breathing. These are great indicators of stress, mental or physical. Awareness brings understanding and the ability to manage.

THE FOUR PILLARS

We can access our body systems through focusing on four aspects in our training - what are usually referred to as the Four Pillars in Systema. These are breathing, relaxation, posture and movement. While the four are, of course, inter-dependent, we can to some extent separate them out for training purposes. We will start by looking at each pillar in turn and suggesting some basic exercises before going on to combine them, add in the use of equipment and working them into some specific topics.

One last thing before we start. Practice everything here in a way appropriate to your current condition. If you have any concerns or questions, seek advice from a medical professional. Don't rush any of the activities, there is no "going for the burn" or any of that nonsense here. Exercise and activities are not a punishment, they should be something enjoyed. Long terms gains over short term pains!

CHAPTER TWO
BREATHING

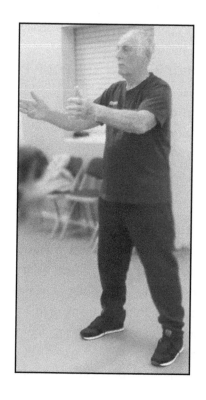

The core of Systema is the simple action of breathing. Breathing is one of the few bodily processes that can either be voluntary or involuntary. It can take place automatically without thinking about it, or we can consciously alter it. This unique relationship between our thinking and our bodily processes, means that breath work plays an important role in our health, particularly when it comes to stress management.

We breathe 24/7, sub-consciously most of the time, and that is where problems begin. Over time, we lose track of our breathing, we lose the feeling of connection between our mind and body. Have you ever wondered how a baby can scream so loudly for so long? Should you try and replicate this feat as an adult, I'm betting you will not only go hoarse quite quickly, you will also run out of puff within a few minutes. The baby's secret is "belly breathing." Babies usually indulge in diaphragmatic breathing, where the belly moves as the baby breathes in and out. We all are born with the ability to breathe in this way but tend to move on to chest breathing as adults, often to even more shallow breathing as we move into our senior years..

Breathing has both a psychological and a physical aspect. When we inhale, the lungs expand, a result of the contraction of the diaphragm and intercostal muscles, thus expanding the thoracic cavity. Upon exhalation, the lungs recoil to force air out. Adults normally take 12 to 20 breaths per minute. Strenuous exercise can drive the breath rate up to an average of 45 breaths per minute.

If we become emotionally upset or angry, our breathing is directly affected. It tends to become more shallow, we may sob, or feel short of breath. Likewise, slowing the breathing can calm the mind. This has been known and practiced for centuries in many traditions, modern science is just beginning to understand and corroborate the mind-breathe-body connection. For example, researchers at Trinity College Dublin showed, for the first time, that breathing directly affects the levels of noradrenaline in the brain. This chemical messenger is released when we are challenged, curious, exercised, focused or emotionally aroused, and, if produced at the right levels, helps the brain develop new neural pathways.

In other words, the way we breathe directly affects the chemistry of our brains in a way that can improve our brain health. The conclusion was that attention is influenced by our breath and that it is possible to optimise our attentions by focusing on our breathing.

Another recent study, at North Shore University Hospital in Long Island, showed that breathing manipulation activated different parts of the brain. These findings support the advice that individuals have been giving for millennia: that during times of stress, focusing on one's breathing can

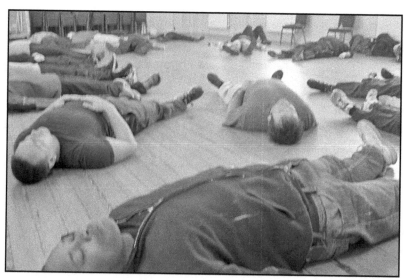

actually change the brain. Exercises involving specific breathing patterns appear to alter the connectivity between parts of the brain and allow access to internal sites that normally are inaccessible to us.

From our "senior" perspective, it may be that we have gotten out of touch with our breathing and it has consequently become more shallow and less attached to our activities - so we find ourselves getting increasingly short of breath doing even the most everyday of tasks. It may also be that we have some condition which restricts our breathing. In these cases we may also need to strengthen our breath function in order to regain our full capability. The first step for all of our work is to practice conscious control of our breathing.

BREATHING LEVELS

Breathing can be practiced almost anywhere and by anyone. Having said that,

there is one caveat - always be aware of you blood pressure, particularly when doing breath holds. If at any time you feel you blood pressure rising, come straight out the exercise, take some Recovery Breaths i necessary (see later). If you do have blood pressure issues, always check with your Doctor before trying anything new. Appropriate breathing exercises should help with the condition but always work under medical advice. I advise that you take your time with these exercises. Although we present them all here in one block, they should be practiced over a period of time, in a progressive way. Do not move on until you are comfortable with the previous method. Unless otherwise directed, all breathing for these exercises is inhale nose, exhale mouth.

Let's start with something simple. Sit or stand comfortably and just become aware of your breathing. Don't take a deep breath, don't force anything or do anything "special." Just "feel inside" and notice the sensations of inhale and exhale. We call this Circular Breathing. Two halves of a circle, inhale / exhale. Both the same length, with a smooth transition between them. A room full of people practicing this always reminds me of the sea coming in and going out on the shore, which itself is a nice image for the breathing.

Once we have that mental connection we can being to control our breathing. At first we will look at the depth. The longer the breath, the deeper we are breathing. We work on four levels.

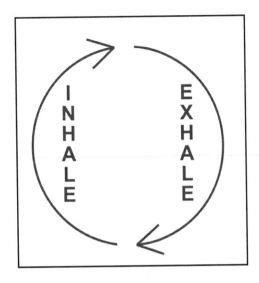

chest expands a little on the inhale and relaxes back on the exhale.

Burst Breathing
The most shallow, this is also called Recovery Breath. The inhale is through the nose, then almost immediately out through the mouth. So the breath only just reaches the top part of the lungs, there is no expansion of the chest. Some liken this method to a dog panting, it certainly sounds similar! Burst breathing is most often use to recover the breath if we are winded, to overcome immediate stress and to bring us sharply back into the present moment. It is generally not done for very long, just long enough for us to recover or stabilise ourselves

Upper Chest Breathing
We can think of this as our everyday breathing, how we tend to be breathing when we are not thinking about it. The

Deep Chest Breathing
This is how we tend to breathe when we are consciously taking a "deep breath." The chest expands more to draw air deeper into the lungs. It's sometimes how people try and breath when they are out of breath, where they would be better served by Burst Breathing.

Belly Breathing
Also known as Diaphragmatic Breathing. This is the deepest of all. Here, the air is drawn into the lungs by movement of the diaphragm. This is the method used by singers, martial artists and others. There are two versions, normal and reverse. For normal Belly Breathing, the diaphragm moves down, sucking air into the lungs. This pushes the belly out. On the out breath, the diaphragm relaxes, air passes out of the

lungs and the belly flattens. For reverse breathing, the diaphragm moves in and up on the inhale, pulling the belly in. On the exhale, the diaphragm pushes down to force the air out, and the belly expands. For both methods, there is not so much obvious movement of the upper chest. However, the lower chest will be expanding, particularly around the back.

Let's go back to our Circular Breathing. Make the circle a little larger and see how the longer the breath, the deeper it goes. No need to work down into the diaphragm yet, unless you are used to that method.

BREATHING SHAPES

For breathing patterns and length of breath, we work with shapes. These are easy to remember and simple to put into practice. Having said that, things can get challenging when it comes to longer breaths and breath holds, so take things step by step. We have already mentioned Circular Breathing. If we add in a breath hold, we get Triangular Breathing. The first triangle is inhale-hold-

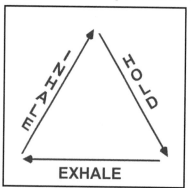

exhale. The sides are equal, so imagine inhale, two, three, hold, two, three, exhale, two three and so on. The reverse triangle is inhale, exhale, hold, again each for the same length.

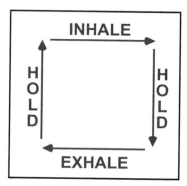

If we add in a breath hold on each side, we get Square Breathing. So, inhale-hold - exhale - hold. Again, each is of equal length. If we change the length, say with shorter or longer holds, we get Rectangle Breathing. So, perhaps inhale for three, hold for six, exhale for three, hold for six - or vice-versa.

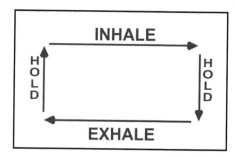

Breathing is a very simple process - we are breathing in, out, or we are holding the breath. But already I hope you can see how controlling depth and "shape" starts to give us a large variety of methods. To start, practice each shape, beginning with and ending with the circle. Keep the length of ach quite short and comfortable to start. The aim for now is to get used to the methods, not to force anything.

BREATHING EXERCISES

Once we have some ideas for breathing methods we can begin to put them into exercises. We will start with some simple Circular Breathing (CB) and look at how we can use it to help manage stress. I think it would be fair to say that most of our everyday stress is in the mind. We tend to be thinking about the future or the past - we worry about things that have happened, or things that may or may not happen in future. CB helps bring us back to the here and now and calms the mind.

Imagine you have a jar, you fill the bottom with dirt, then top it up with water. Put the lid on the jar and shake. The previously clear water will now be cloudy. If we set the jar down, the heavier dirt will gradually settle to the bottom and the water will become clear again. We are using the same principle. If we sit quietly for a time and concentrate only on our breathing, those racing thoughts slowly subside and we will be left with a wonderfully clear mind!

This kind of simple practice can be surprisingly effective, you can come out of it feeling very refreshed, as though you had just had a good sleep. This is because practicing these methods actually changes our brain states - from Beta(our everyday state) through to Gamma (deep, dreamless sleep).

QUIET SITTING

This is our first and easiest method, you only need a few minutes to do it. Sit quietly, close your eyes and begin Circle Breathing. Inhale nose, exhale mouth. Not too deep, remember, keep everything comfortable. Keep the body relaxed but maintain good posture - don't slump. Don't worry about counting the breath, just let it come and go.

Keep the mind focused on the breathing as much as you can and let all the muscles relax. You may find that thoughts spring up - don't fight them, again, just let them come and go. Don't analyse them or get sidetracked by any thoughts, think of them as clouds floating by. If you find yourself drifting mentally, come back to the breathing. Inhale, exhale.

When you are done, slowly open the eyes and bring yourself back into the world. You may wish to stretch or move around a little before resuming your activities.

LADDERS

This is a method of learning to control our breathing and so put ourselves into deeper states of relaxation, or to make our movement more efficient. We simply give each breath a specific length, gradually

EXHALE	■	■	■	■ ■
INHALE				
EXHALE	■	■	■	■ ■
INHALE				
EXHALE	■	■	■	
INHALE				
EXHALE	■	■	■	
INHALE				
EXHALE	■			
INHALE				
EXHALE	■			
INHALE				

increasing, then coming back down again. Imagine climbing a ladder, the rungs get further apart. We reach the top, the climb back down.

I suggest at first trying 2-4-6-8-6-4-2. Begin CB and count inhale 1-2, exhale 1-2. After a time, increase to inhale 1,2,3,4 exhale 1,2,3,4. Next work up to a six count, then to eight if you can. After a while on 8, go back down to 6, then 4 and finish on 2 The main thing is to keep the counting consistent and the breathing smooth. Also, the depth of breath should match the length. A 2 count is quite shallow, 8 uses deep chest breathing. How long you spend on each number depends on how much time you have, the top number you go to depends on how slow you can breathe! As always, never force, build up slowly. You may find at the first your upper number is quite low but over time you will go up into double figures quite comfortably!

Once you have the idea you ca work it into your Quiet Sitting. A the count increases, you will fin yourself going into deeper level of relaxation. Counting also help maintain focus.

It is easy to put Ladder Breathing into movement or exercise. I walking, for example, we count b steps. So inhale for four steps exhale for four and so on. Again the speed should be consistent Go up the ladder and back down. Once yo have done that, settle on the count that yo felt most comfortable on. Usually around the 4-6 mark for me. Walk while maintaining tha speed. You will find it helps increase endurance and you will be able to go fo longer distances without feeling tired. O course, you can also try this with other types of movement or exercise too.

DEEP BREATHING

If we need to work a little deeper, we can use Diaphragm Breathing to really slow down both mind and body. This is a longer exercise than the Quiet Sitting, so you will need to set aside a little time. You may also want to change your environment to suit – dim the lights and so on.

Lie on your back on a flat surface (or in bed) with your knees bent. Place a pillow under your head your knees for support. Place one hand on your upper chest and the other on your belly, just below your rib cage and above your navel.

Now begin Ladder Breathing. Once you get up the higher numbers, breathe in slowly through your nose, letting the air in deeply, towards your lower belly. The air going into your nose should move downward so that you feel your stomach rise with your other hand. The movement and airflow should be smooth, you shouldn't feel like you're forcing your lower belly out. The hand on your chest remains still, while the one on your belly rises up.

Next, let your belly relax. You should feel the hand that's over it fall inward. Again. don't force your stomach by clenching. Exhale through the mouth. The hand on your belly should move down to its original position.

At first, just do this for a couple of minutes at a time. The diaphragm is like a big muscle, if we over-use it it will become a

little sore and tender! Over time, you can extend the length of the practice.

If you would like to work with Reverse Breathing, start from the same position. This time, on the inhale, draw the abdomen in and up, pulling the air into the nose. Again, the hand on the chest should not move very much. For the exhale, push down and out, squeezing the air out as the belly expands.

Keep the mind focused entirely on the breathing and the physical sensations - the rise and fall of your hands, the movement of the belly. Let all the other muscles relax, imagine you are sinking down into the surface beneath you. The breathing should naturally lengthen as you go on. Do not be tempted to rush straight into super-deep breaths, let them grow naturally.

Once again, should you find your thoughts wandering, bring the focus back to the breathing and movements. When you are

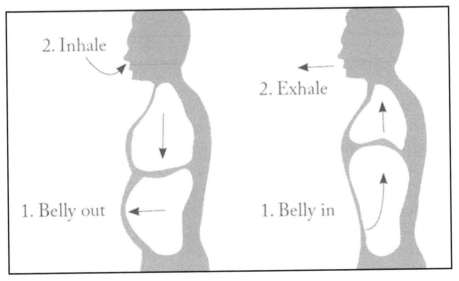

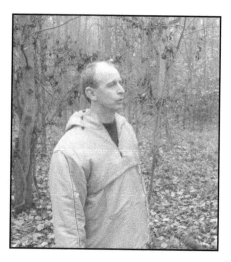

indicator of overall health. Besides this, breath holds can improve lung capacity, develop focus and will power, increase your anaerobic threshold and help us to manage fear and tension.

This practice should be carefully monitored and practiced incrementally, though. Most people can hold their breath for a minute or so with no training. You may be interested to know that free-divers (people who hold their breath at depth underwater) can hold for over ten minutes, a remarkable feat of will power and self control.

ready, slowly come out of the state by shortening the breaths a little, bringing the breathing back up into the chest. Think of it in the same way as you fall asleep and wake up, usually gradually. In fact, it is not uncommon for people to fall asleep while doing this exercise, which is why we advise you leave plenty of time to do it! As such, it's also a good method to use if you are having trouble sleeping at night.

Once done, get up slowly and stretch / move around a little before returning to your regular activities.

When you come out of a breath hold, you may want to try and fill your lungs with as much air as possible. Avoid the temptation, instead go into the Burst Breathing we mentioned earlier. This will bring you back to stability much quicker. It's a little like the advice given to people who have water after wandering in the desert for a few days - don't gulp, take little sips!

FEAR CONTROL

BREATH HOLDS AND RECOVERY

The breath holds in our earlier shapes are relatively short. It is also possible to practice them as a separate thing, though. For this, simply inhale or exhale and hold! Make sure you are somewhere comfortable when you do this and if you begin to feel light headed, stop immediately. Some say that the length of the breath hold is a good

Being unable to breath is a primal fear, perhaps our most primal. Using breath holds, we can bring this fear into the body in a controlled way and so learn how to manage it. Sit comfortably and begin CB. After a time, take an in breath and hold. Try not to overfill the chest, inhale to around 80% capacity. You will at some point feel a fear or tension, maybe in the chest or solar plexus. Relax it either by doing some movement, or just by calming the mind.

This feeling will return. Again, try to relax it and continue holding. At some point the need to breath will be overwhelming. When it is, start breathing again, but go into Burst Breathing. Remember, shallow, panting breaths. Gradually increase their length and depth until you are back to normal. Then repeat the same, holding on an exhale.

I can't stress how important it is that you do this work slowly and carefully. If you have any adverse effects, or if you suffer from blood pressure or similar issues, always check with your Doctor first. However if you do this work I'm sure you will very quickly feel the benefits, both physical and psychological. Because that "fear feeling" we experience during breath holds is pretty much the same that we experience during a stressful incident. As soon as you feel that fear /tension, work to get rid of it as you did during the exercise. You may even use some Burst Breathing to help, if appropriate to do so.

PYRAMID

This combines the Ladder method with the Triangle, Rectangle or Square. Let's use a Square Pyramid as an example. We run through the same progression, two, four, six, eight, etc but this time add in a breath hold too. So that is inhale for two, hold for two, exhale for two, hold for two, then on to four and so on. We are now practicing not only lengthening / deepening the breath but also working the holds too. Of course, you can add this in to your walking or other activities too, always with the caveat of it being to safe to practice breath holds in the circumstances.

That covers our foundation breathing methods. Although it may only take ten minutes to read, there is already a huge amount of work here. So please just start with some CB and gradually work up from there- you don't have to do all of these at once!

Above all, breath work can be carried out whatever our physical condition. We may be a little frail and lacking mobility, we may even be bed bound. We can still work these breathing methods - in fact I'd say that it becomes even more important to do so.

Because part of overall health is our mental health. It is very easy to get despondent when we are experiencing health problems. We may focus on the negative. Breathing gives us at least one thing to hold on to, to take control of. From this we can begin to exert a positive influence on our emotional state and, hopefully, begin to appreciate the things we are still capable of. It is also important to keep the mind active if the body is less mobile, something we will talk about more later on.

CHAPTER THREE
POSTURE

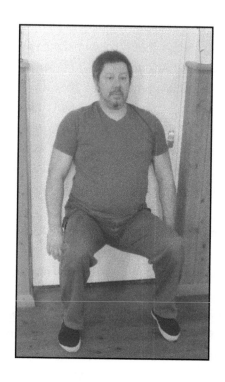

Our second pillar is posture. We can think of posture in terms of our body being a machine that is working efficiently and effectively. Picture a car engine, everything is engineered to be the right size and be in the right place. Add even an inch to the length of an axle and there are problems!

When it comes to the human body, the problem is that over time even just gravity will have an effect on our posture. Then there are poor habits and lifestyle factors, injury or illness and also psychological issues. Because one thing with posture is that it is often a reflection of our internal state. Angry people grimace, raise their shoulders and so on. Sad people slouch and look down. On the beach some of us pull our bellies in as attractive people walk past! If our "out of sorts" emotional state becomes the norm, it will have a powerful impact on our posture. So let us first determine what "good posture" is, check to see if we have it, then look at some ways of regaining it if we haven't.

What we consider "good posture" is to have the body upright and balanced. Stand in front of a full length mirror if you have one. Try facing it and then turning sideways and run through this checklist:

HEAD - does it protrude forward or tilt back?

UPPER BACK - is it hunched or curved?

SHOULDERS - are they lifted up around your ears? Is one higher than the other?

LOWER BACK - is it arched?

ABDOMEN - does your stomach stick out

HIPS - do they push forward? Is one higher than the other?

KNEES – do they point inwards? Is your weight more on one leg than the other?

FEET – is your weight on the outside or insides of the feet? Do your toes point out?

If you are of an age and can answer *no* to most of the above, then well done! For most of us life will have taken its toll. If we are very sedentary it is likely that our upper back slumps a little. If we carry something heavy on one shoulder a lot, it is likely that shoulder is higher than the other. If we like our food and beer it is likely we have a bit of a pot belly going on.

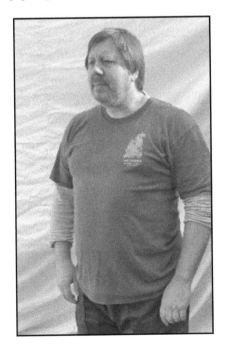

And as I mentioned before, it is said that gravity compresses the spine over the years to the extent of losing us at least two inches in height! Luckily these things can all be fixed. Of course, if we have suffered an injury then there may well be more permanent consequence to our posture. What we have to be aware of is how we compensate for the issue in another part of the body. For example, it's quite common for people with a bad leg to develop a problem in the opposite hip – it's doing more work now.

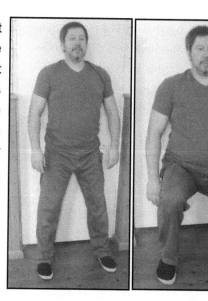

POSTURE TEST

In a book such as this it is difficult to give ideas for every ailment or condition but we will do our best to give you a comprehensive overall guide, some ideas on specifics and give you a good start should you choose to take up a type of therapy or movement regime that will help. So having carried out a visual check, let's get physical.

Stand barefoot with your back against a flat wall. Your feet should be about shoulder width apart and around ten inches away from the wall (adjust position to suit.). Squat down a little - there's no need to go too low at this stage. This is what we call an Assisted Squat position. Now we run through a checklist again.

HEAD – can the back of your head touch the wall without tilting?

SHOULDERS – can they both touch the wall equally?

LOWER BACK – can you press your lower back to the wall so that there is no gap? You can check with your hand. Try tilting the hips up slightly to help.

KNEES – are they pointing forward and in line with the toes?

If you can do all of the above then you have good posture - the spine is straight and slightly lengthened, the head is upright, the shoulders and hips level. How does it feel? Note where any tension or discomfort shows. This indicates an area that needs to be worked on.

Now work the same procedure sitting in a char – a high backed chair is best, rather than an armchair! Head upright, back straight, spine lengthened, feet flat on the floor. If you can, stay in each of these

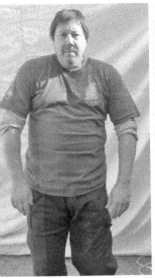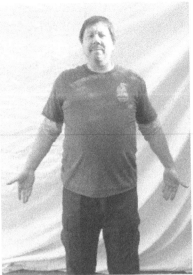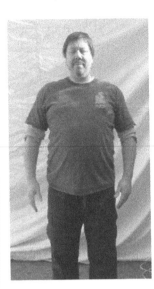

positions for a few minutes. In Systema we work a lot with "feelings" rather than visual structure. The latter can be useful but we find that our bodies learn best through feeling. Once we experience good posture, our body can recognise when we are in or out of it. So take the time to adopt the above two positions for a few minutes every day. Relax into them (without slouching). This isn't about standing to attention, it's about softening the body back into its natural form. Look how toddlers stand, they usually have excellent posture. That's what we are aiming to regain, we just have to help our body to remember! That is our first step. Now, let's look at some specific exercises we can practice.

Stand with your hands at your sides, palms turned out. Pull your shoulder blades in together, as though you are squeezing something between them. Now, keeping the shoulders back, relax them and the arms. Allow your palms to turn so that the palms are now in, thumbs facing forward. This should un-round the shoulders. Don't take them too far back and create tension. After a while you can simply rotate palms out to palms in to get the same position.

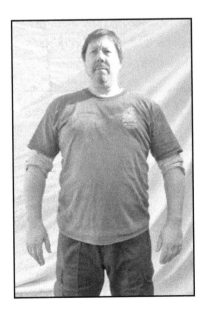

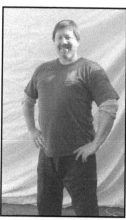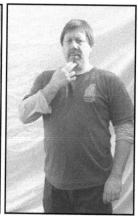

Lift up the ribcage a little. You can move it into the space created by bringing the shoulders back. Do not arch the back, just increase the space between ribcage and hips. Also avoid puffing out the chest, it will raise naturally.

Tighten the abs a little. Pull the belly button in towards the spine. Be sure that you can still breathe comfortably!

Tuck the chin in a little – tucked, not tilting. Now imagine there is a chord coming out of top of your skull and someone is gently pulling it. This should have the effect of lifting the head up.

Keep the feet roughly shoulder-width apart. The knees and toes should align. Wiggle the hips gently side to side, allow them to settle into a level position. Be sure your backside is not sticking out. If anything, tilt the pelvis a little by tucking the tailbone in. This will lengthen the spine downward.

You may try doing all of this in a sequence. You may just work one or two. I find I use the head and shoulder alignments a lot during the day if I am sat at the computer for hours on end. Prevention is better than cure!

ACTIVITIES

As we mentioned, posture is not fixed and needs to adapt to the circumstances. There are a few obvious examples of this, particularly in context of this book.

Lifting

If we have a strong core then we can maybe get away with poor posture when lifting a heavy object. Actually, not even heavy, sometimes it is the size and shape of the object that is the issue. People tend to bend at the waist, grab the object, then straighten up.

Put simply, when we bend forward we are switching off the lower back muscles. We then quickly fire them up again on straightening, with the added load to lift on top. This is what can cause twinges and spasms. It doesn't have to be a load - you'd be surprised at the number of men I know, of a certain age, who twinge their backs while putting on trousers, socks or doing up their shoelaces! The same conditions apply.

Where possible, then, bend at the knees to lower the body. Grasp the object and stand. In effect, we are doing a squat, which allows the back to remain straight and the

thigh muscles to deal with the load

Sitting

When sitting for a prolonged time, particularly at a desk or table, it is easy for our posture to slip. First of all, check your chair and desk. Are both at a suitable height? Next, check your general position. Can you place your feet flat on the ground? Or, as I do, you may find a footrest helpful. I also have a back support on my office chair which also helps prevent slouching.

A while ago I found I was getting a very stiff back down one side after sitting for a while. I was sitting on an office chair that had wheels, and I found that as I was leaning forward a little onto the desk, the wheels were moving back slightly. This increased my lean, and was also making me twist a little, hence the back pain. I now have a chair with a fixed base and have everything lined up so I can sit looking forward.

If your are sitting in an armchair for a long time, then see if you can use a cushion or a bolster for support. Again, you might find raising your feet up on to a rest or stool helpful. Every now and then, wiggle your shoulders and straighten your spine. Above all, try not to hunch or slouch forward. This will only put pressure on your lungs

and digestive system. If you have a stick by your chair, raise it above your head now and then, or try some of the exercises in our later chapter.

Whether you are sitting or standing, always check your posture when using your mobile phone. It is very easy to get "drawn in" to the screen, with a corresponding slump in posture. Holding the phone up a little higher will help.

Sleeping

We spend a huge amount of time in bed but often pay little attention to how we sleep. As far as posture goes, the main thing is to check your mattress and pillow. Both should be firm enough to give support but comfortable. The size of pillow may vary a little depending if you sleep on your side, front or back.

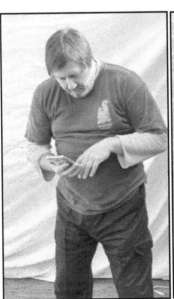 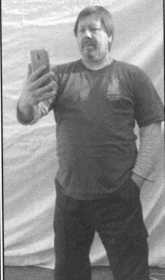

You may find it useful to place a pillow or small bolster under you lower back or under / between your legs. Get into your normal sleeping position and picture your spine. Is it straight, or does it dip and curve anywhere? That place is where you may need some support, be it a bolster or, perhaps, a new, firmer mattress.

If you are bed-bound, then be sure to have good support for when you are sitting up in bed. Specifically designed pillows are available and are probably better than bunching up a few cushions behind you. Be sure to have everything you need within easy reach so that you don't have to stretch or twist to reach it.

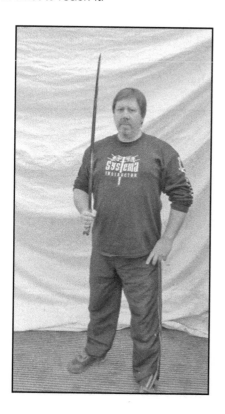

SWORD / STICK

We will be looking at using a stick in more details later on, but we shall finish this chapter with a look at how even just holding a stick can help with posture.

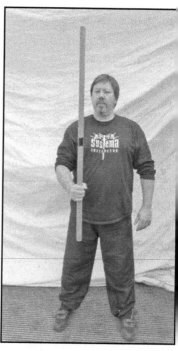

Well, I say stick but in Systema this exercise is usually carried out with a sword! If you have a sword to hand, then fine, if not you can use a stick, preferably one with a little weight to it.

This is more of an internal exercise. Our first corrections to posture where largely done by observation. We now need to take the feeling from those earlier exercises and work them on a deeper level.

Stand upright and hold the sword / stick out in front at waist height. Keep the hand fairly close to the body. Now run through our earlier check list - head, shoulders, spine, etc. Keep the stick upright and imagine the spine in the same position. Take a few breaths and release any undue tension. Wriggle the body a little if necessary. Now o beyond the surface level and feel eeper into the body. Often, we carry ension in some of the smaller, support muscles. Inhale, exhale and release. Feel where you might need to make any small adjustments to your structure. Spend a few minutes doing this, gradually allowing the posture to settle in place.

The sword or stick should remain still once you are settled. Think of the object as the needle of a compass - it will flicker a bit at first, then settle at North. So any imbalance or instability in the body will be reflected in the stick.

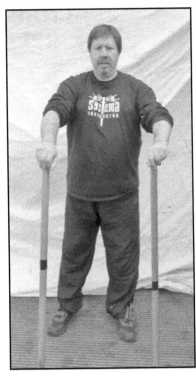

Another option is to use two sticks. Place them a foot or so in front and rest your palms on the top of each stick. You shouldn't be putting any weight in the stick, just let the hands rest lightly. Now run through the same procedure. As before, any imbalance in the body will cause one or both sticks to lean. Settle the body and they will stray upright.

These are some simple exercises for checking and regaining posture. As we go through, we will add in some extra work, particularly with sticks, that will also aid good body posture. Naturally, everything we do affects everything else, so breathing and mobility rely on good posture but in turn make good posture easier. As you will see later on, this means that just by doing one exercise we can be working more than one of our Pillars or body systems. Of course, we can't stay completely upright and get into a car, for example. However, our natural resting position should always be as described above. These are simple exercises but may be challenging in some cases. Always take your time, I emphasise again how important it is to *relax* into these positions rather than force them. So let's move onto to our next Pillar and find out how we can release excess tension.

CHAPTER FOUR
RELAXATION

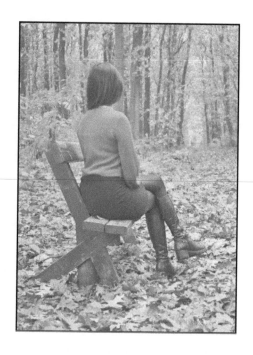

Our third Pillar is the feeling and understanding of tension / relaxation within the body. As we age, we tend to accumulate tension, for all the usual reasons. However, barring injury or medical condition, there is no biological reason that we should suffer from high tension levels. As we mentioned before, stress is often, though not always, primarily an emotional issue. In that respect, we have already taken the first steps by understanding how we can use breathing to calm the psyche.

But let's now also tie that into our physical work. We know that the mind and body are closely linked, with the breath acting as a bridge between the two. Mainstream exercise in the west usually centres around the physical - do some movements, count, build up a sweat and so on. A more layered approach, such as is seen in Systema, recognises the deep connection between emotional and physical and works to strengthen that connection.

During lock-down (still in it in the UK at time of writing) a "celebrity" put out a free series of exercise routines on TV (as though fitness professionals across the country weren't already in enough hardship!). I watched one and was dismayed, even angry to see the kind of exercise he was promoting, particularly for the elderly. No warm up, no breathing, nothing about posture, just lots of fast, ballistic movements to get you out of breath. In fact, I heard of at least two people who injured themselves while doing one of his routines. Highly irresponsible, but sadly indicative of what the mainstream thinks exercise should look like. Frankly, I wouldn't even show this to young people, there is so much potential for harm.

But what do we mean by "relaxation"? It tends to conjure up images of reclining on a sun-lounger with a cocktail to hand! Nothing wrong with that, but our meaning is something a little different. What we are referring to when we talk about relaxation is using the minimal amount of muscular and mental tension to carry out a task. That task may be as simple as standing still! It is interesting to see how some people think they have to engage so many muscles in order just to stand. In fact, our body is largely supported by our skeletal structure. When properly aligned it supports our posture perfectly well, with need only for a little tension here and there.

Excess tension creeps in from many reason. Fear is usually the culprit. If we fear falling, we tend to clutch at something for support, which, ironically, usually makes us more prone to falling. If we are surprised, the muscles tense in anticipation of danger.

Of course, the fear may also relate to an injury or condition. If a part of the body is injured, we try and protect it with tension, or at least hold it back from moving. It is interesting, though, to note that we do the same thing even when the injury has healed.

The body carries a memory of everything that has happened to it. The more dramatic the event, the deeper the memory is stored. This is where Systema comes into its own as a healing art. Because when we relax deep into the muscles, those "memories" will be released along with the physical tension, making this a powerful form of emotional healing too.

At the base level, though, we are monitoring the body for excess tension and working to release it. Tension is insidious. It creeps up on us and, if we are not careful, gradually becomes part of our everyday movement, as we discussed when talking about posture. Let's first try operating with tension to get a feel for it.

Try doing a few squats with every muscle locked tight. Go slow! There is a chance your blood pressure will rise and your movement will most likely feel inhibited and uncomfortable. Or we may say it feels *unnatural*. In Systema we talk a lot about natural movement. Watch how a cat walks, how a monkey climbs, this is all part of their activity, they don't "exercise!" The same with children, they have great natural movement. This is something we want to regain, to get back to and relaxation is key.

SELECTIVE TENSION

Our first exercise uses selective tension to teach us how to feel where tension is in the body and how to release it via our

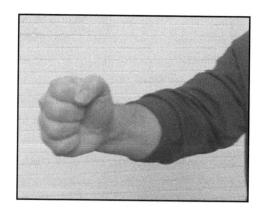

breathing. It works by tensing selected parts of the body on an inhale, holding it in for a short time, then releasing the tension on the exhale. Let's practice with a hand. Sit comfortably, take an in-breath, it doesn't have to be too deep and, as you do so, clench your fist. Hold the breath, hold the tension in place for ten seconds, or so. Now exhale slowly and uncurl the fist as you do so.

That's all there is to it! There are a few pointers we need to bear in mind. The first is that the breath and the physical motion must be linked, they must be working at the same time. So the speed you clench your fist follows the speed of the breathing. In your mind, count, 1,2,3 as you inhale, the fingers move at the same speed. Ditto with the exhale, 1,2,3, uncurl the fingers. Of course, the breath can be longer or shorter as required but the internal / external link must be in place. This way we condition the body to relax more on every exhale.

The second pointer is that the tension is selective - it must only affect one part of the body. So if we are tensing the arms, for example, the rest of the body remains relaxed. To help with this, we being by tensing large parts - the limbs, the shoulders, etc. Later on, we can work down to muscle groups, or even individual muscles. Let's run through the whole routine.

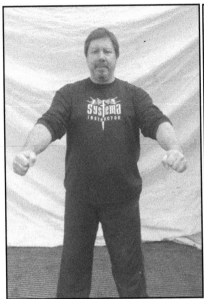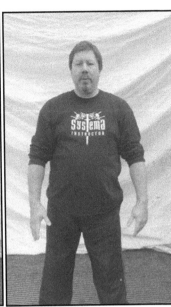

Lay down or sit somewhere quiet and comfortable. Go into Circular Breathing and just let body and mind relax. We will start in the feet. When ready, inhale and tense the feet, exhale and relax. Do this three times. Keep breathing depth and speed comfortable. Next work all the way up the legs, so feet, calves, thighs and butt. Remember, everything else stays relaxed. Repeat three times.

Next follow this sequence, inhale tense, exhale relax, three times. Work just the abdomen, back, chest, shoulders, arms, head/neck.

To finish we apply the tension to the whole body, head to toe. Slow the breath a little, inhale, tense, hold. Exhale, relax, hold. Repeat this twice. On the third time, tense and hold for a little longer. Now, when you exhale do it as a burst breath and release the tension quickly - *PAH!* Stay where you are for a minute or so, have a stretch, move around a little before getting up.

You don't have to go through the whole sequence, you can just work a couple of parts. This is particularly useful if, during the day, you feel some tension creeping in. Use the ST procedure on that area to stop it taking hold. In this way the exercise also works as a diagnostic tool - we can use it to scan ourselves for potential problems. Of course you can vary length of breathing, depth or tension and number of repetitions to suit, too. This is a simple exercise but one that we do in almost every training session, it is so valuable on many levels. If we return to our Posture exercises, should you feel tension in a specific area, use this method to release it.

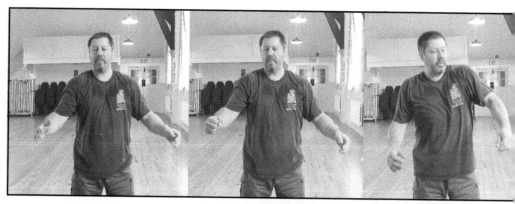

Let's say you are standing against the wall and your left shoulder is stiff. Inhale and increase the tension in that shoulder. Hold it in tight as you hold the breath, for at least twenty seconds if you can. Now slowly exhale and let that tension go with the breath. Repeat as necessary.

MOVING TENSION

The ability to move tension through the body is a useful skill. In Systema we use this as a method to absorb powerful blows and strikes. It works equally well in moving tension away from a stiff shoulder and out of the hand, too! Another benefit of this exercise is that it teaches us about "movement chains" within the body, how parts of the body connect in order to transmit movement, what we refer to as Wave Movement. However that is moving away from our current topic, so, back to tension!

We are going to start by tensing the right hand into a fist. Next, tense the forearm,

the upper arm and the shoulder. Maintain the tension for now, taking it across to the other side, shoulder, upper arm, forearm, left fist. At the end, both arms and shoulder are tense, all on the inhale.

Next, exhale, start to relax, left fist first, left forearm, upper arm, shoulder, then across and back down to the right fist. In effect, this is the wave tension exercise, but only across the arms.

Once you can comfortably do that, it's time for stage two. The sequence is the same, only this time as the forearm tenses, the fist rel

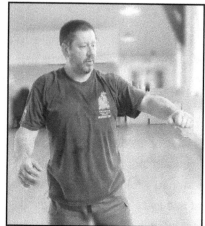

axes. As the upper arm tenses, the forearm relaxes and so on. All the way across, until the left fist tenses, then relaxes, releasing the tension away. The tension, then, is moving, it passes through each muscle group without leaving anything behind.

Think of it a ball of tension that moves from the right hand to the left. The breathing pattern is inhale right fist to right chest, exhale left chest to left fist. This may take a while for you to get but stick with it. Once you have the idea, reverse the direction, left to right. You can also work the same method with the legs - foot, calf, thigh, butt and across.

Once you are able to do this, you can start to link any two points of the body together and practice moving the tension between them - right foot to left hand, for example. The ability this develops will allow you to move any unwanted tension out of the body. Let's say you have a stiff back - inhale and tense it up, exhale and see if you can "move" the tension out through the foot. This principle also works well with the sort of tension that comes from shock or fear. You can almost "shake it away" with this method.

RELAXING THE MIND

That takes care of muscular tension, though it should have a calming mental effect also. But what it we want to work deeper into relaxing the psyche? For that we can work a deeper version of Quiet Sitting by adding in another layer - visualisation. You may have heard the expression "I'm off to my happy place," well this exercise shows you how to build your own!

In essence a Happy Place is a calm space, a mental construct that we can retreat to in times of stress. That may be in response to something that is happening. I last used this method when in the dentist chair for root canal treatment! Or it may just be that you want a bit of time away from it all. Here's how it works.

The first thing is to create our space. The physical requirements are the same as our earlier breathing exercises, seated or laying down in a comfortable position. Close your eyes, begin Circular Breathing as before and let mind and body settle down. Next, I want you to think back to a happy time and place. I like to think of the time I was sitting on a lovely beach in the Med.

Once you've established the place, work through each of your senses. In the case of the beach, feel the warmth of the sun on your face. Listen to the whisper of the sea as it gently laps against the short. Smell the sun-tan lotion, the tang of salt in the air. Gulls call in the background, a faint, cooling breeze ruffles your hair. Paint the scene in your mind, make the colours bright and vivid, the sensations real and pleasant.

Now we are immersed in our scene, we

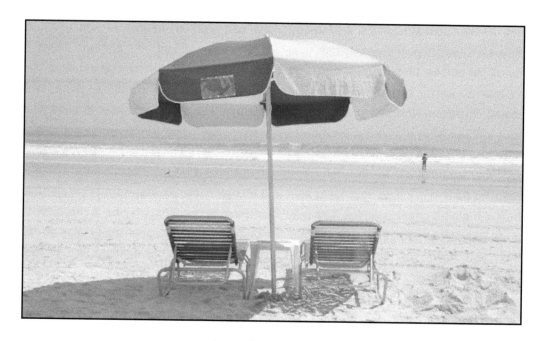

need to anchor it in our memory. An anchor is an impulse (stimulus, trigger) which causes a specific response, which is always the same. In contrast to a reflex, this response is learned and not hereditary. The basic principle was discovered by the Russian neuro physiologist Pavlov during his famous experiments with dogs. Anchors can occur in all sensory systems, for example a certain smell may trigger a very specific memory.

For the purpose of this exercise, we will choose a physical anchor, something very simple but definite. We will make fist with one hand, but tucking the thumb inside the fist rather than outside. Now squeeze the fingers, putting pressure on the thumb. Do this a few times, with each squeeze your scene becomes more and more vivid in your mind.

To finish, slowly come out of your vision and back into the real world. Take a couple of minutes as before to stretch and move around before resuming your activities.

The anchor can be any movement or action similar to the above. It is best to choose something that is not an everyday movement, something a little unusual. Your visualisation can be of anything, it doesn't even have to be a real experience. You might imagine singing on stage with your favourite group, or flying high through the clouds on the back of an eagle! A powerful image is to take a scene from our childhood, a happy experience that we can remember and re-live in our minds. As long as you can make that initial visualisation as vivid and real and possible in your mind, involving all he senses, it will do the job. When you need to go there, trigger the mental state by using your anchor movement.

It might sound strange, but this is a surprisingly effective method. Our imaginations are much more powerful than we think and, as we have already established, what goes in our mind has a profound effect on our body. Boring or unpleasant situations may never be the same again!

THE BEACH VISUALISATION

Picture yourself walking along a lovely, sunny beach. There is no-one else around.

Hear the gentle hiss of the waves on the sand as you inhale and exhale.

Your feet sink into the warm sand. Wiggle your toes. Feel the warmth of the sun on your skin. Let your muscles relax.

A cool, refreshing breeze ruffles your hair. You hear the distant gulls. You smell the salt air, and suntan lotion.

Ahead, is a sun lounger. You sit in it and recline into the soft padding. Paint the scene in your mind, make the colours bright and vivid, the sensations real and pleasant.

Relax and sink back into the comfortable lounger as the waves and your breathing become slower.

Feel the energy of the sea. Feel how you connect to that energy. Your breath is the wind and waves.

Each time you exhale, let go of something you don't need. Worries, stress, tension, all flow away into the sea.

Rest for a way, safe, warm, relaxed.

When ready, stand and walk back along the beach they way you came. Before leaving, take a last look around at the scene. Remember, this place is always here for you, you can visit it at any time.

To finish, slowly open your eyes and come back to the here and now.

CHAPTER FIVE
MOVEMENT

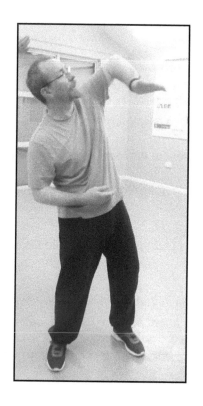

The final Pillar is movement and this really comprise several things - mobility, co-ordination, balance, self-awareness, and so on. To start, we will look at mobility in terms of our range of motion. This relates to our joints. When we are young, our joints are free and soft, as we age they can tend to stiffen up and get a bit rusty!

As we mentioned before, children explore their world through uninhibited movement. As we age we get fixed into movement patterns. We sit at a desk all day, sit on a bus, then sit and watch TV all night. Our range of motion (ROM) decreases, simply through lack of use. Imagine a garden gate not opened for a couple of years - it is bound to squeak when you then try and open it! For movement then, it is very important that we maintain our ROM throughout the body.

We will start with a head to toe joint rotation routine that is very simple to practice and also acts as a safe way of developing our ROM. It is always important not to force the joints, in fact, first of all we will work well within our comfortable ROM.

These exercises can be done standing or sitting. You can run them through as a whole routine and/or do a couple of them during the day as you need to. It is important that any joint rotation work is carried out with no tension, so you may wish to run through the Selective Tension exercise before this one. If a joint does feel particularly stiff or tense, or you have an injury or condition, then never force the movement. Just work within your comfortable ROM. If you can get a little movement, that is better than nothing. Medical advise for specific conditions aside, always move where possible. If something is a little stiff, don't be tempted to leave it and never move it, the condition will then not improve.

If you feel any sharp or sudden pain then immediately stop the movement and seek medical advise. Always proceed with care and caution, especially if you have not exercised for some time.

Our standard procedure is to start with linear movements. If we take the shoulders as an example, we first lift the shoulders straight up and drop them. We then move the shoulders back and forward. Use the linear movement to pinpoint any areas of tension. If everything is okay, go on to the circular movements - in this example by rotating the shoulders.

In some cases we will give specific inhale/exhale patterns for the movement, but the main thing is to keep the breathing natural and smooth. The amount of repetitions is up to you, a few is usually enough , though if you have a particular area of stiffness you might wish to spend a little more time on that. We normally start with the head and work down, or you may wish to start with the shoulders if they are particularly tense.

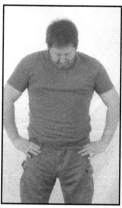 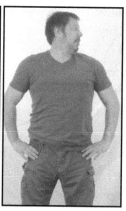

Stand straight, shoulders relaxed. Inhale. Exhale and let the chin drop forward as far as is comfortable. Inhale and bring the head upright. Exhale and tilt the head back as far as comfortable. Repeat a few times. Next, from the same start point, exhale and turn to look left. Inhale to the centre, then exhale and look right.

If everything is okay, slowly rotate the head. Drop the chin down and circle the head, again just going as far as you are comfortable with. Keep the breath natural and slow. After a few circles, change direction.

Now for the shoulders. Inhale and lift the

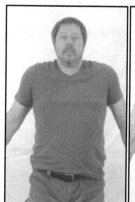 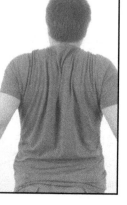

shoulders up, exhale and let them drop. That is our vertical line. Next, inhale and squeeze the shoulder blades together, exhale and bring them forward - imagine you are trying to touch the shoulders together at the front. Repeat a few times. If everything is okay, then begin to rotate the shoulders, circle them back and forth. Keep everything relaxed, breathe naturally.

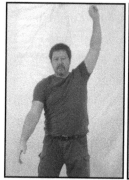 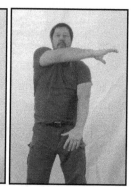

Next, some larger movements. Stand with hands at your sides. In turn, lift each arm up above your head. Then lift each arm out to the side, shoulder height if you can, and make big circles with the hands. Go backwards first, then forwards. You can rotate each arm separately, or both together, in a swimming-type movement. After that rotate the arms in front of you, like a windmill. After a while, change direction and reverse the circle. On all of these exercises, try not to turn the trunk when rotating the arms.

We next move down the arms into the elbows. Place your hands out at chest height and bend each elbow in turn, bringing the hand back towards the chest.

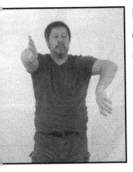

From there, circle both elbows out in front. You might like to imagine you are conducting an orchestra! Keep the shoulders relaxed.

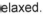

from side to side, without moving the hips. You may find there is not much movement at first, don't worry. After that, with the hips still again, make circles with the chest. Now repeat the same movements with the stomach, then the hips - back and forth, side to side and circle. When rotating the hips, be sure to keep the knees relaxed and not locked in place.

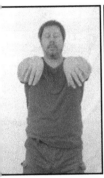
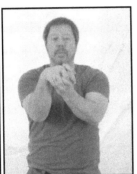

The hands are next. Hold them out in front and flex the wrists up and down. Then shake the hands a few times and make circles with the wrists. After that, wriggle the fingers and open and close the hands a few times. Finally, link the fingers together and roll the wrists.

After that, we work into the trunk. Place hands on hips and push your chest out, then back. Next, sway the chest

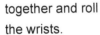
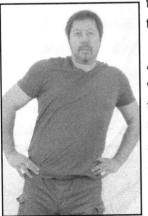

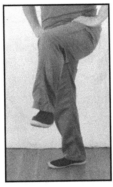
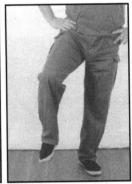

We finish with the legs. You can work some of these sitting or standing, with support if required. Lift a knee up and down, swing the knee back and forth a few times. Then flex the ankle. Place the foot down if you need a rest. Now lift again and allow the whole leg to swing back and forth from the hip. Everything should be relaxed. From there, progress into rotating each join in turn - ankle, knee and hip. Imagine you are drawing an expanding circle with the toes. Repeat with the other leg. If doing this as a whole routine, we like to finish with an all over shake!

Having worked through our joints should give us a good feel for our ROM. Work on areas

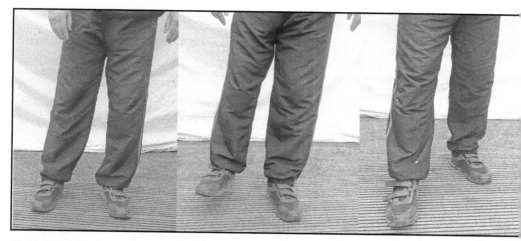

that need it, in conjunction with all the previous exercises. Remember, if you find your movement getting stuck, check that you aren't holding your breath.

WALKING

The most common form of movement for most of us is walking. We learn to do this as kids and then rarely, if ever, think about it again! As with all our other pillars, this means that bad habits creep in, so I find it really does pay to spend some time on walking. In fact, we have classes where we might spend up to an hour just walking. I say just walking, of course we are doing specific things, not just ambling around the hall!

The first thing is to check your walk. This may be a little difficult - a full length mirror at the end of a corridor may work! If not, get a friend to observe you, or, better still, have them film you walking on their phone or camera. You can go through pretty much

the same points as our earlier posture check. Look also for how you step - is there a limp or hesitation? Do your feet splay out as you walk? Do you lead with head?

Systema walking is based on the pendulum principle. In that respect it is closer to some forms of dance than the crouching "moving from the centre" stances seen in most Oriental martial arts. This means that our stepping should be light and lively.

If we think back to our earlier posture points, that is a good start. Stand up, bring the shoulders slightly back and lift the ribcage. The head is suspended from above. This should already give us some "lift." Now, put your weight into one leg. Relax the hip and just let the other leg swing for a bit. When you've had enough of that, bring the foot to the floor, transfer the weight across and swing the other leg. This is how relaxed your legs should be when walking.

The next question is how we lift the leg and how we place the foot down. The first, we do

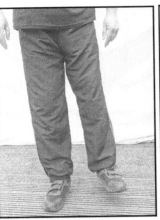
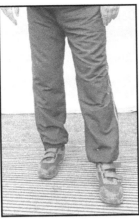

walk all over again - well, it is! In class we call this waddle the Charlie Chaplin walk. The hips are swaying as we move, the upper body stays upright and light. There should be very little impact with ground. One good test is to walk across a wooden or squeaky floor, making as little noise as possible. I'm no lightweight but using this method can glide quietly across even a resonant floor.

not by engaging the thigh muscles, but by rotating the hip up. Stand as before and imagine you are a gunfighter from the old West! Place the hands ready to draw your gun but instead of reaching for the gun, bring your hip up to the hand - lift and rotate it towards the hand. As you do see, be careful not to tilt the body. Rotate back to lower the foot.

The next step (haha) is to look at the foot. People usually push up from the foot onto the toe, move the leg forward, then fall into the heel. Indeed, some people call walking "controlled falling." We are going to glide, making our walk not only smoother and more efficient but also less wearing on the joints. Go back to rotating the hip. Try and lift the foot all in one go. In other words, the sole of the foot remains parallel to the floor the whole time. Same for placing the foot down, the sole contacts the floor equally.

Once you get the idea on the spot, try taking a few steps. You may feel that it is quite awkward and a bit like learning to

Practice a little each day. Over time the movement will become less obvious and more subtle. You may find yourself using muscles that have not been used for a while, so don't over-do it. Also remember our other pillars, breathing, posture, relaxation. For an added challenge you could balance a book or similar on your head, a good test of our abilities! Once you have the idea of this method, start to gradually incorporate it into your everyday movement. Glide from the kitchen door to the kettle, for example! The same goes for our earlier ROM exercises - roll your shoulders as you put a coat on or off. If sitting, lift a foot and do some ankle rotations. As before, little and often is the key!

MOVING WITH RELAXATION

Most of us have experienced moving with tension at some time in our life. If you twisted an ankle, for example, you know what it is to limp. Part of the body is held in tension away from the floor in order to protect it. But it is not just physical tension that affects our movement, emotional tension can too. If we get angry or aggressive, typically the chest swells, the hands are raised the heart rate increased and so on.

As usual, in isolation, or for a short time, this is not an issue. Where such behaviour becomes normalised, though, is where problems begin. Our movement deteriorates as a result, people can even end up hunched completely over or severely restricted in their mobility. One way to counter this is to always think about moving with or into relaxation. When we walk, our body should feel light. Everything we do is with that feeling of lightness, smoothness and flow, like a well-oiled machine or a cat! Moving in such a way makes it much easier for us to go into "flow state," or what athletes call "being in the zone." Research has shown that these states are when we are out our happiest - everything just happens naturally, nothing is forced or tense.

Much of Systema training is about accessing our flow state. In terms of movement, here is a routine that will get you started, we learn to move to release tension.

Stand normally and turn your head to one side as far as you can. At some point you will feel tension in the neck muscles. When you do, turn the body in the direction you

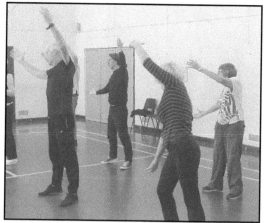

are facing, exhale and walk a few steps. In other words, you release the tension by turning into it and walking. You should walk until the body naturally stops, normally just a few steps is all that is required. Repeat a couple of times on each side

From the same position, twist one shoulder back as far you can. Again, when you feel the tension, turn and walk to release, on an exhale. Repeat on both sides. Try the same with both shoulders - pull them forward or back, then step to remove the tension.

From there, work into the chest. Stick it out in front, as though being pulled by a string from your sternum. Exhale and move forward, releasing the tension. Repeat from the back, pushing the shoulder blades out.

After this, reach out with a hand. Twist and stretch as far as you can, then allow the tension to pull your body forward to release it.

ext work from the hips. Push the hips out one direction, then let the feet step in rder to release the tension and re-align e body.

inally, work from the feet - as with the ands, stretch a foot out an then let the ody follow. In each of the above, try and xhale on your movement.

Once you have the idea, you can be working on a more subtle level. Whenever ou feel some imbalance in the body, exhale, move into it and allow the body to naturally re-align. Over time, you will find you can achieve the same result with less obvious movement. In this way, we begin to fine tune our body into reacting to tension with appropriate movement.

At time of writing, one of our students mentioned something that happened to him. He had been lifting a heavy weight and felt his back twinge alarmingly. He had not quite got the right posture when lifting. Rather than push through it, he immediately let the weight down, sharply exhaled and dropped prone to the floor. Now, it might seem like a strange reaction, but doing so prevented a twinge from becoming something far more serious.

Try and make it a habit, then, to move into relaxation. Think about how you get up from a chair, for example. The usual procedure is for people to lean forwards, place hands on thighs and push up. Instead, try keeping the spine straight and imagine being pulled up from the crown of the head. You will find the body rises with much less effort and a feeling of lightness. Try the same when going upstairs, or any other even slightly stressful movement.

If in doubt, when you feel stuck or under tension, change your breathing. To learn how to do this, go into one of the core exercises. Let's say a push-up. From start position, exhale. Then inhale and very slowly lower. As soon as you feel tension in the arms, exhale and complete the move. Do the same thing on the upward movement.

You can try this on any exercise, the point being as soon as you feel tension, change the breath, ie inhale of exhale. This should help release the tension. Bring these methods into your everyday activities and feel the flow!

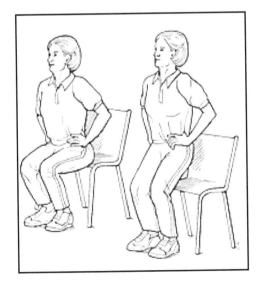

CHAPTER SIX
CORE EXERCISES

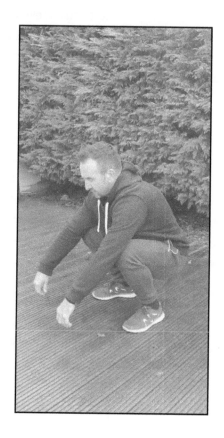

We will now move on to Systema's core exercises. They are called this for two reasons. One, they are all about exercising and strengthening the core components of the body - the legs, torso and upper body. But also because these few simple exercises form the core method of bodyweight training, and more besides.

This means that unlike some martial arts, we do not need to learn long series of intricate moves. In Systema, we can gain much of our functional movement from the core exercises. They also provide us with the bulk of our solo training methods, meaning that we can train without a partners. Furthermore, due to Systema's unique Four Pillars approach, the exercises are also good for our health.

Three exercises may not sound like much, or it may sound a little boring to always be doing the same thing. But this is the genius of the Systema founders. By using the Four Pillars as our variables, there are countless tweaks and variations on the basic movements - enough to challenge us on every level but within our own framework. It is also possible, of course, to make the exercise less challenging, so we have a method we can use if we are not in top condition or have some issues. That is where we will start - with what we call "assisted" methods of each exercise. Then we will show the standard version, plus some variations that you might like to try. But please be sure you have the basic movement down first. While these exercises are simple, to do them properly is quite a challenge!

As we mentioned, the Four Pillars are present throughout. Initially, that means keeping a focus on good posture, being aware of any excess tension, moving slowly and with breathing. We will show some specific breathing patterns, later on you can experiment with these. Be very aware as you practice of any unusual pain or discomfort and also keep and eye on your blood pressure, particularly during squats. Any issues, come out of the exercises immediately, regulate your breathing and, if needed, consult your doctor.

SQUATS

Let's start with the squat. The basic position is to stand with feet shoulder width or so and slowly bend the knees, sinking down as low as you can to the floor. From here, we straighten back up again. In other words, a movement we do every time we sit down! Some call the squat the *King of Exercises*, and with good reason. It works the largest muscle group in the body, trains balance and co-ordination, aids digestive health, strengthens our stabilisers and works our cardio system and metabolic rate.

Our first step is the assisted wall squat. We have to some extent covered this in our chapter on Posture, we need only make a slight tweak to that exercise. Place your

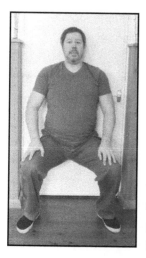

back to the wall as before, feet out in a comfortable position. There are two major structural points to check with a squat. The spine should be as straight as possible (even if there is a lean, the spine should be aligned and not curved.) And the knees should always align with the toes. Imagine a line coming out from your big toe - the knee should point along this line. If the knee is inward or outward from this line, then it becomes load bearing rather than load transferring, with the risk of damage.

So, once in position against the wall, check to see you have good contact with the spine and that the knees are not bowed. Now, slowly lower yourself down. If you can, move until your thighs are parallel to the floor. If not, go to your limit and hold there.

Maintain the position, breathe, relax. You may experience some discomfort in the thighs. This is because your thigh muscles are now taking your bodyweight rather than your back muscles. Breathe that tension away. When ready, straighten the knees and return to the start position. If you need some help getting back up, "walk" up the wall with your shoulders, or use a stick or similar for support.

Now try the same thing as a movement. Take an in breath. Exhale and squat, inhale and come back up. If it helps, imagine the body emptying and relaxing on the exhale. Then use the inhale to pull the body back up, as though inflating from within.

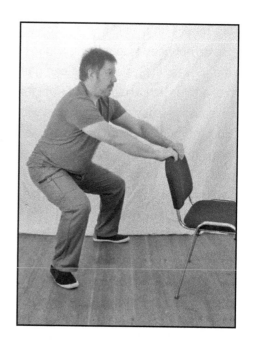

Another way to practice the assisted squat is to use something in front of you or to the sides as support. This might be a table or kitchen counter, it might be a pair of chairs. This method is particularly good if you have a knee injury. After many years of kung-fu low stance abuse, I rehabbed my knees with this method.

Hold your support and make sure it is firm enough to take whatever weight you need to put on it. Bring the feet out to comfortable

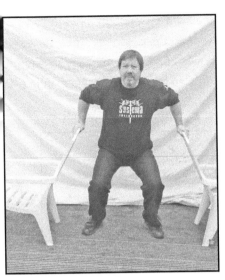

Holding this posture for a while will also help relax the hips and keeps the legs "loaded" without so much strain as a squat. In may places around the world, this is a common sitting or resting position. It is also a good way of transitioning to and from the ground, more on that later!

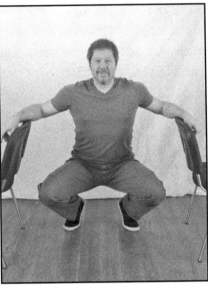

osition, take a moment to check your tructural alignments. Inhale. Exhale and ink. Hold the posture and take some reaths. Check your knee alignment again. Jse you support to keep some weight off f the knee. This allows you to strengthen he knee without putting too much strain on . When ready, exhale to raise again.

As before, then work continuous squats. Take your time, nice and steady, work with he breathing. Every now and then check or tension in the shoulders and hips and also your alignment. Work as may reps as you feel comfortable with. No need to work o failure, in fact it is rarely beneficial to do so.

Another option to ease into squats, or as a good exercise in its own right, is the Cossack Squat. In this, we drop down again, but this time the heels are lifted off of the ground. You can work into it in the same way, with support, if required.

Once you can do the assisted version, try working solo. Have some support to hand if required. You may find that you can't sink as low when standing free, but that is okay. It is far more important to maintain your form than distorting it to go a bit lower. For breathing, start with exhale down, inhale up. Match the speed of your movement to the breathing. Keep an eye on the alignment of the spine and also the knees. If you get a lot of tension at some point, just stop there, don't try and push through it.

What you can try, is go back to the wall and sink to that point where you felt the tension. Hold this position. Inhale and tense the leg muscles as much as you can. Hold for 20-30 seconds. Exhale and release the tension. Try this a few times, then go back to the unassisted squat.

PUSH UPS

Everyone knows Push ups, or at least thinks that they do! However it is rare to see push ups performed correctly. Let's start with the assisted version.

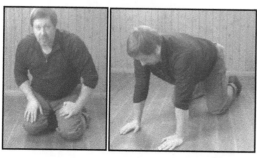

We begin in kneeling position. Lean forward and bring the hands to the floor. Shuffle the feet back and put the knees onto the floor.

Before you begin hold this position. Check that your back is not slumped or hunched up. Think of the back as a table, it should be level. The hands should be under the shoulders, or a little wider. Make

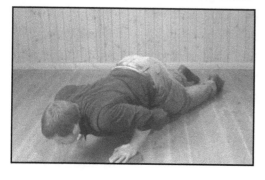

sure they are far enough forward to you t lower comfortably. Inhale. Take an exhal and slowly bend the arms. Try to keep th shoulders as relaxed as possible. Inhale an come back up again.

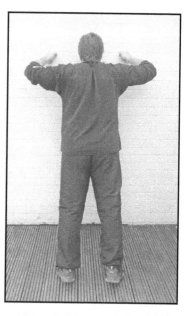

You can work a similar method against the wall. Place palms on the wall and bring the feet back a little. Now lower to the wall and push back. Again, check alignment and tension, inhale, exhale.

From the previous table position, we can work another great exercise to strengthen our core muscles. Get in place again, the hands and feet should form the squares of a rectangle. Inhale. Now exhale as you slowly lift one hand and stretch it forward. You should remain stable while in this position, with three points of support on the floor. Inhale and return the hand to the floor.

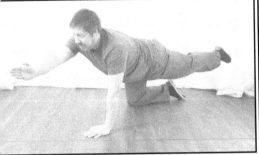
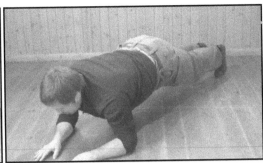

Repeat with the opposite hand.

Now do the same thing with each leg. Stretch each out in turn on an exhale. Finally, extend the opposite hand and foot on each side. Each time, you should feel the body core activating.

The next step is to work a static push up, what is known as a plank. Start on the knees again, place the hands down. Now raise the knees and straighten the legs. From there, bring the weight forward onto the elbows. Check the back as before, keep it nice and level. Hold, keep the breathing working and try to relax the body without letting it sag. When you are ready, lower slowly to the floor.

For a variation, try a side plank. Lay on one side, with the feet stacked. Push up from the elbow and rest on the forearm. Keep the body straight again and don't let the hips sag down. The final version is the full plank. Now we rest on the hands, in push up position. Check structure, keep the hands under the shoulders and maintain the position with minimal tension. Don't forget to breathe.

How long you hold each of these is up to you. The key point is to release any excess tension, via breathing or via a little wriggling. A short hold is fine at first, you can build up over time if you wish. Again, do not train until failure, always rest when you need to.

From the last position, all we have to do to go into full push-up is bend the arms. Inhale down, exhale up. The body should go all the

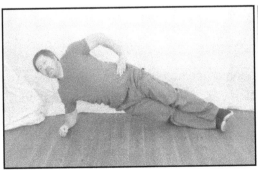
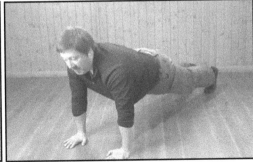

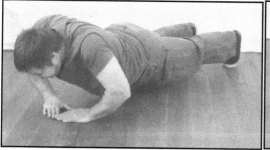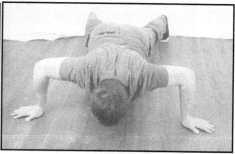

way down to the floor as one unit - no bobbing! Keep the movement slow and smooth, in time with the breathing. Work with the palms down at first.

Systema push ups are usually done on the fists - for alignment and other reasons. You might find this uncomfortable at first, so practice on a soft surface. Rather than pushing yourself up, imagine you are pushing the floor away with your fists. Make sure that the fists are positioned directly under the shoulders, keep the body straight and try not too engage the shoulders too much. Once again, inhale down, exhale up, smoothly

position of the hands and/or feet. Close together, wide apart and so on.

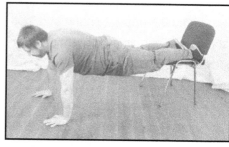

Elevate the feet using a chair or similar for more of a challenge. Or, from the normal position, as you lower on the push up, move one knee towards the elbow, then back again as you rise.

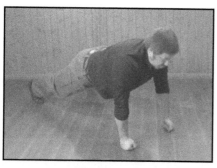

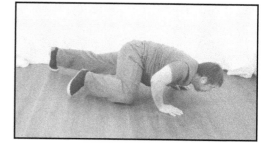

There are many more variations once we have the basic movement down. If you feel capable, here are a few ideas. Adjust the

Another method is to start with the hips up high. As you lower the arms, the body "swoops" down, forward and up. Then return to the start position.

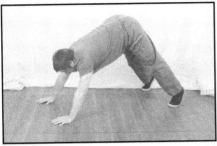

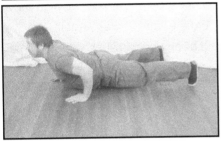

ground movement and mobility training. Let's start with something simple.

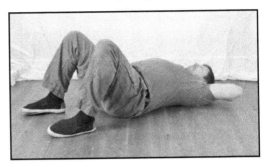

These are just some ideas. When you start working with the breath, you can add in even more variations, as we shall see a little later on.

The simplest version of the sit up is a crunch. Lay on the floor, knees raised, hands behind the head. Inhale, then on the exhale lift the head up towards the knees. You don't have to lift very far. Inhale, return to the start

SIT UPS

Sit ups are a great way to work the central core but I would advise that you take extreme care with these exercises if you have any back problems. In fact it may be best to avoid certain movements altogether, depending on your condition. Always be guided by your health care professional.

We start on the floor for sit ups. This gives us the advantage of having much more support, so it is usually easier to maintain good posture. These exercises also form a good base for any future work we do on

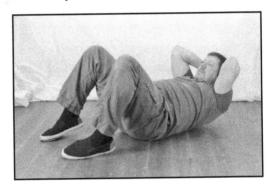

position. You can experiment with lifting the feet and/or bringing the knees in as you lift the head too. Make sure to keep the back pressed against the floor.

For the next exercise, lay back, with arms at sides. Inhale, then on the exhale slowly lift one or both feet about a little off of the ground. Inhale and lower. An alternative is to raise the feet and then hold them in place. Use burst breathing as you hold, then lower slowly, Try to keep the body as relaxed as possible.

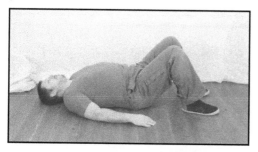

Another way to work into and strengthen the core is to lay on your back with knees up, feet flat. Inhale.

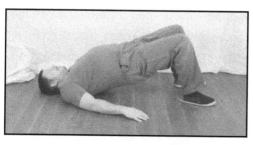

On the exhale, raise the hips up. Be sure to keep the body straight, do not twist the hips or shoulders. Inhale and lower to the floor again.

We can also work the lower back. This time we lay on our front, with the hands on the back of the head. Exhale. On the inhale,

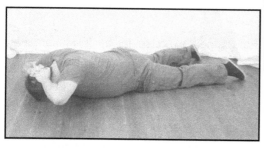

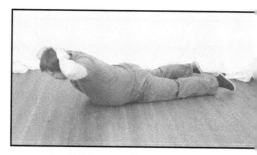

left the chest off of the floor as high as you can. Exhale and lower. Again, be very mindful of any back issues with this type of movement.

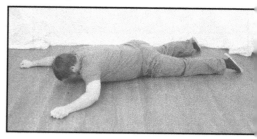

A variation on the above is to have the hands and feet splayed out. Exhale. On the inhale, lift the body again and raise the hands and feet up - as though you are doing a parachute jump! Exhale and return to the start position.

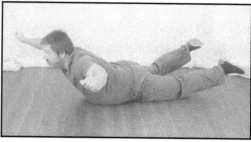

The next exercise is what we call a Circle Up. It uses the momentum of a rolling movement to perform a sit up. This makes

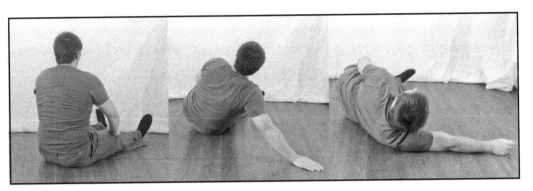

it less strain on the back and abs and is also a good foundation exercise for learning to fall and roll. It also teaches us how to use the legs in order to assist ground movement. As we are contacting the ground, you might like to work on a soft surface at first, such as a carpet or mat.

We start the exercise in a sitting position, with the back nice and straight. Keep the legs relaxed throughout. Allow the body to fall to the right and slightly back. The right hand can contact the floor, but be sure not to brace the arm. Instead, allow the hand to slide away from you, so bringing the side of the body smoothly to the floor.

Next roll across the shoulders, you can use a slight rotation to help, exactly the same as our earlier Joint Rotation exercise. Come onto the left hand side and use a little support from the left arm to continue the roll into an upward movement. The momentum takes the body up and you return to the start position. Repeat in the same direction a few times, then fall to the left.

If you find it difficult to sit up from the side position, then bring the knees up towards the chest at that point and kick the feet out. This will give you some extra momentum and should help bring the body upright.

You can practice this method in one direction, or work falling right, then left and so on. Whichever way you, get used to exhaling on the fall and roll, inhaling on the

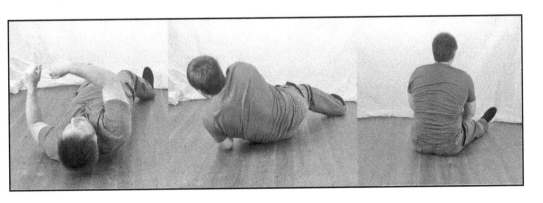

lift. Keep the body as soft as you can and be sure not to bang the elbows in the floor - keep you movement smooth and, as always, breathe!

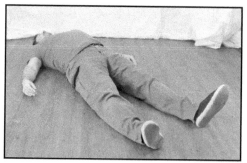

Let's now progress to the full sit up. Start position is to lay flat on the floor. Keep the body and particularly the legs as relaxed as possible. You may find at first that tension in the legs makes you lift the feet in order to bring the body upright. Again, if you do find the move difficult, draw the knees in and kick the feet out as before.
Ideally, though, we need to be activating the core muscles to perform the movement.

Inhale, then exhale and sit the body straight up. The spine should remain straight all the way through the movement,

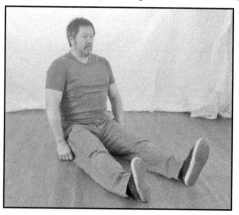

do not slouch. Keep the arms at the side, again in order to engage the core fully. Inhale and sit back.

We also have a static sit up, equivalent to the plank. From the start position, bring the body up to an angle of around 45 degrees. Maintain this position for while, say a count of ten to begin with. Then, slowly lower back down again. When static, keep the breathing working - you may wish to burst breath to help the body stay relaxed. You can also experiment with holding the body at greater or lesser angles.

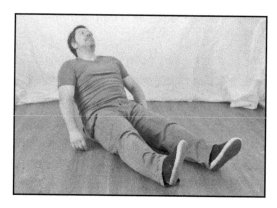

Our final version of the sit up is the leg raise. I will again add a note of caution in here for anyone with back or neck issues. Also, if you are not used to this type of movement I would advise getting good at the basic sit ups before trying the leg raise. The key, as always, is to work step by step, establishing your comfortable range of motion to start with.

From a prone position, inhale. Then, as

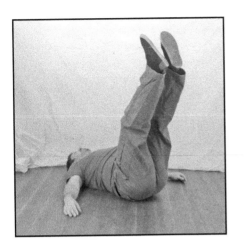

you exhale lift the feet directly up and over the head. If you find this tough at first, you can try starting from a sitting position and letting the body fall softly back. As you do so, use the momentum of the fall to lift your legs. Bring the feet over as far as you can. In time, you may be able to bring the toes right down to the ground.

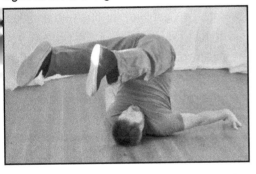

The bodyweight should rest on the shoulders, not the neck! See how the hands can also help with support. F r o m here, inhale and return to the start position.

COMBINATION AND FLOW

These then are our core exercises. As with the breathing, you can read through all this in ten minutes but there is months of work here! Take your time and go steady, always with an eye to health.

A conventional approach to exercise is to use the numbers approach. You write up a list of say, ten pushups, squat and sit ups, rest for a minute then repeat. Do the exercises as fast as you can, because we need intensity! Systema takes a different approach. As mentioned before, we prefer to think in terms of activity rather than exercise.

There is nothing wrong with setting yourself set numbers of movements. But think of them all as part of one routine or movement. Think about it - you don't break up walking into the kitchen and making a cup of tea into component parts, you just do it. We find that this approach introduces the concept of *flow* into our movements and also makes it much easier to map our "exercise" movements into our daily activities. This is doubly important as we age, as it is this type of natural movement that helps keep us healthy and active. So let's take our core movements and see how we can build a "flow routine" with them.

We will keep the speed fairly slow to start. If you wish you can of course speed the movements up but at first we always advise working at a steady pace. Of course you can also go the opposite way and slow these movements down as much as you can - another challenge! Start in standing position

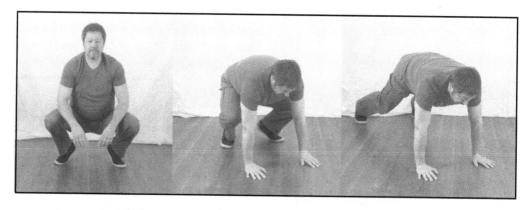

and first go down into a squat, standard or Cossack. From here, bring the hands to the floor and slide the feet back.

and do a push up. From the plank position slide your feet forward into a squat and repeat the squat.

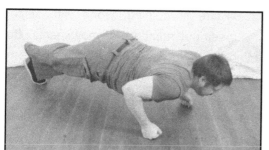

Now do a push-up. Lower the body to the floor and roll over onto your back. Next do a sit up. Lay back on the floor and do a leg raise.

You can cycle this movement round, or you can repeat each movement within the cycle as many times as you like. The point is that the transition between each movement becomes a movement in itself. We don't stop the squat, take a glug of water, then get into our push up position, everything is integrated. Of course, you can do any of the variations of each exercise too. Remember to breathe correctly throughout! Keep the movements in line with your breathing and work at a steady pace. Take your time!

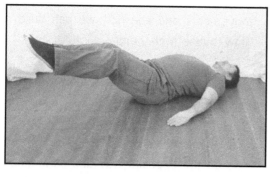

Next, repeat the sit up. Roll onto your front

Once you have this idea I hope you can see how to apply it to all the movements we describe here and from there integrate them into your life. Need to pick something up off the floor? Don't bend, instead breathe and squat! Look for opportunities to do these movements, don't regard them as "punishment" exercise.

BREATHWORK

So far we have described the basic inhale/exhale pattern for the core movements. We will finish this chapter with looking at how we can add in our earlier breath-work, particularly through the use of our shapes.

Circular Breathing is our start point - inhale down, exhale up, or vice versa. If you want to work breath holds in, then start with the triangle. Let's use push ups as our movement.

From push up position, exhale. Inhale and lower down. Hold the breath and push up. Exhale and lower down. Hold the breath and push up. Of course you can switch the pattern, for example - Inhale and hold. Lower down. Exhale and push up. Hold and lower down. Inhale and push up.

Then you can work Square. Inhale down, hold up, exhale down, hold up and so on. Go into Rectangle by varying the lengths of breath or holds.

Let's look at Ladders next. We will apply to squats to give our arms a rest! Get into standing position. Inhale down, exhale up. Now inhale up and down, exhale up and down.

After that, inhale over two full squats, exhale over two. Then three. From three, we go back down the ladder, two, one, then inhale down exhale up. Of course you can go up to whichever number you like, as long as it is within your capabilities. Naturally you can reverse the breathing too. The point is that our breath becomes longer and deeper with each rung - and be sure to check that the tempo of the movement remains constant, no speeding up!

You can work this method purely with breath holds. Stand ready, inhale and hold for one squat. Exhale. Inhale and hold to two squats. Exhale. Inhale and hold for three. Exhale. Now inhale and hold for three squats. Exhale. Inhale and hold to two squats. Exhale. Inhale and hold for one squats. Exhale.

In every case, particularly where you are using breath holds, be sure to recover, with Burst Breathing if required, between each set of movements. Take your time on this part, one of the purposes of this exercise is to teach you how to manage and recover your breathing / mental state / nervous system.

Working with breathing patterns opens up so many variations on our core movements. I highly recommend you seek out the downloads and books put out by Vladimir Vasiliev on this topic, there is a wealth of information available to guide you through this important and highly rewarding work.

CHAPTER SEVEN
STRETCHING

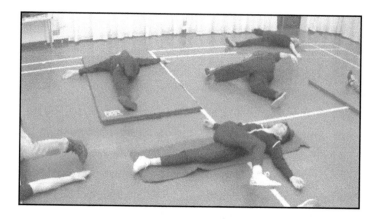

Stretching is a great exercise, particularly as we age. It can be done slowly in increments, there is no strain on joints, and we are usually working on the floor, so have plenty of support. In fact, medical conditions aside, there is no reason we should not be as "flexible" later in life as when we were children. Indeed, there are many example on Youtube and other places of people with great flexibility even into their 80s.

However, mention stretching and people often conjure up images of people tying themselves in knots or holding impossible looking positions. However the Systema approach to stretching is more about releasing tension in the muscles and so restoring our natural range of motion. Mostly, we are looking to overcome something called the *stretch reflex*. The stretch reflex is the contraction of a muscle that occurs in response to its stretch. It is an automatic response that is transmitted to the spinal cord.

In effect, it is the body trying to protect itself from a dangerous movement. Take an arm and move it back and back, at some point the muscles will tense to stop the movement, to prevent the arm from going so far it tears muscle or ligaments. This is good in some cases! However an issue arises when our natural range of motion minimises, particularly as we age.

We tend to settle into fixed patterns of movement. Over a period of time, these become our new norm and anything that takes us beyond that is flagged up as "dangerous." Here's an example. Imagine that you never lift your hand above your head. Over months and years, your body comes to accept that this is an odd movement. The muscles used in that movement may weaken. The body no longer recognises this "shape." So, five years on, you decide to suddenly raise your hand up above your head. The movement is flagged up, and the muscles tense to stop it. This is one way that people get strains, particularly in the back. In fact, you are perfectly able to raise the hand above the head, you have to use the brain to over-ride the reflex.

This is what we are doing when stretching, then. We overcome the SR and allow the muscle to real and lengthen - we all know that a tense muscle is contracted. This lengthening allows our body to move fully once more. This can be achieved quickly, using more intense methods, but here we will focus on gentle ways to dissolve the tension, centred around the breathing, of course!

From out earlier work on Selective Tension, we know that we can release muscle tension with the breath. We apply the same method here. We will do it in one of two ways, moving and static.

For the moving method, we get into position and inhale. We then exhale on our stretching movement. Hold for a few seconds, then inhale as we return to the start position. Repeat as required.

There are two static versions. On the first, we exhale and move into the stretch as above, but then we hold the position, typically for at least a minute. As we hold we use Burst Breathing and focus on relaxing the muscle under tension. Release on an exhale and slowly move back to start position.

For the second version, we exhale and hold position as above. Take a few breaths, then inhale and consciously tense the affected are as much as you can. Hold the tension, hold the breath, for 20-30 seconds at least. Then exhale and release the tension. You should find the muscle relaxes. In effect, we are overloading the are with tension so that the muscle has to let go.

When it comes to stretching movements, there are hundreds, if not thousands! For sake of space we will give you a good set of general stretches here, upper and lower body. You can develop your own or check out other resources for further ideas - always with an eye to safety, of course. Above all avoid any "bouncing" movements or any sudden changes of direction. Slow and steady is best, once again! Should you feel any sharp or sudden pain, immediately come out of the stretch and get checked.

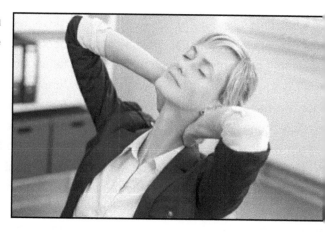

STRETCHING ROUTINE

The movements that follow can be practised as a whole routine or I would encourage you to do them throughout the day as you need to. For example, if you've been sitting for a while, get up and do a few arm stretches, remember, prevention rather than cure!

Some stretches may be more challenging than others, depending on your current condition. Work these with particular care and, as before, let this work seep into your daily activities. Use that reaching up to the high shelf in the supermarket as an excuse to stretch!

The format I generally use with these movements is this - three moving and one static stretch. So we repeat the moving stretch three times, inhale/exhale, with a brief hold in the stretch position. On the first movement, we go only to the first point of tension. Say we are lifting the leg - I will lift the leg on an exhale just as far as it wants to go. On the second and third I might lift or pull it a little further as the muscle relaxes. On the fourth move, I hold in position and breathe. As the muscle relaxes more I may increase the stretch a little. When ready, I exhale and slowly release the stretch - and I emphasise the word *slowly* here!

We are working solo versions of the stretches here but there is nothing to stop you working them with a partner. Here, you help the person get the limb in position and apply whatever pressure is required. This often means we can work deeper into the stretch. However, always be very aware of your partner's levels of tension and comfort. Always release (slowly) when asked to. Be sensitive - and it is best to have a good grounding in the solo methods first, this will help. So, we shall begin with the head and work down.

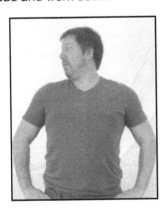

Think back to our rotation exercises where we turned the head. Do the same move but now with an emphasis on relaxing and lengthening the big muscles at the side and back of the neck. Remember, three moving and one static. Turn left and right, then drop

the chin down. After that, drop the head sideways, as though you are trying to touch the shoulder with your ear. Some people like to place a hand on the had and apply pressure with this movement, that is up to you. If you do, pull lightly and remember the aim is to lengthen the opposite side, so pull away from the opposite shoulder rather than down.

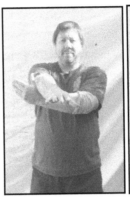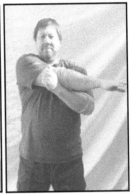

Next, the shoulders. Hold one arm out in front, supported under the elbow. The movement is pulling the arm across, with the aim of opening out the upper back.

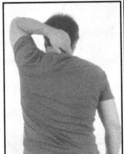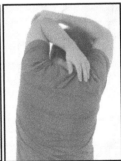

Place one arm behind the head. Reach over and take hold of the elbow and pull it across.

From the shoulders, we work into the trunk.

As always, take care on the bending exercises. Be sure to keep the lower back straight and when lifting up, lead with head - take the head forward and up to lift rather than working from the lower back.

Cross the hands in front of the chest, right hand outside. Inhale. Exhale as you rotate the right palm up, the left hand moves down. Push the hands up and down. Inhale as the hands cross, repeat on the other side.

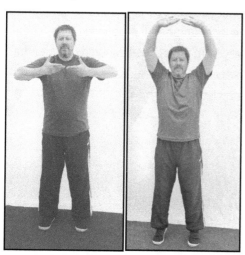

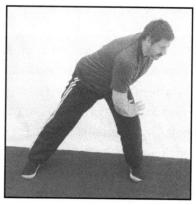

Begin with arms at the waist, palms up. Inhale. Exhale as you rotate the palms and begin to raise them. Push the palms up as high as you can but be sure to keep the shoulders relaxed. Inhale as you circle the hands back to the waist.

Bring your feet out a little wider and place the hands on the hips. Inhale. Exhale and bend, bringing the let hand to rest on the right knee. Push the hips back a little and keep the spine aligned. Inhale and, leading with the head return to the start position. Repeat on the other side.

From the same stance, cross the arms over your chest. Inhale. Exhale as you bend forward. Just go as far as comfortable and

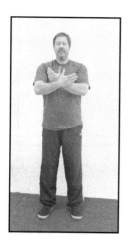
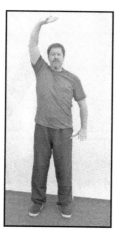

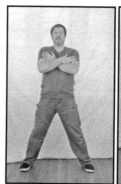
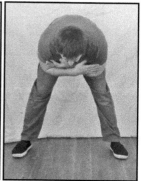

o not slouch. Again, lead the up and down movement with the head. From the same start position, exhale and bend back as far as is comfortable.

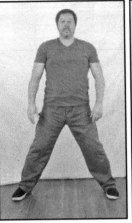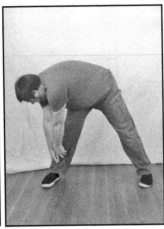

Hang the hands at the sides. Inhale. Bend at the waist and exhale. Reach down and grab the right leg. Inhale and return to start position, then repeat on the left.

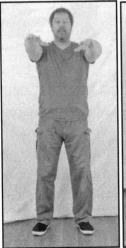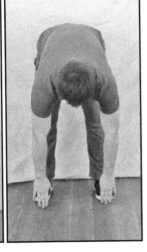

Stand with feet at shoulder width, raise the hands to shoulder height. Inhale. Exhale as you bend at the waist. Reach down as

far as you can, stretching out the lower back. Lead with the head. An alternative to this move if you don't want to fully bend is to use a table or similar for support. Place the hands on the table for support and keep the back at 90 degrees. Push the hips back a little to lengthen out the spine

Having worked the upper body, we now move down into the legs. For most of these stretches we are on the floor. Be sure to have a comfortable surface to work on. Also take care in how you get down to the floor - we will show you how to do this safely later on. Of course, you could work many of these laying on a bed or couch too. We only show one side here, but remember to work both legs. We will start with a preparation exercise.

Lay on your back with legs out, arms at the sides. Inhale and pull your feet in towards

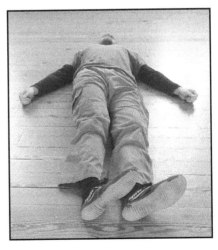

your backside. Exhale and "throw" the feet back out, with the legs as loose as you can make them. Repeat a few times. From the same position, inhale and pull the toes back towards you. Exhale and relax. Next, inhale as you move the feet to each side, exhale as they return to upright position. Think of the feet as windscreen wipers!

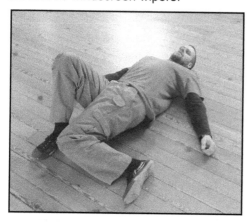

Bring the feet in, raising up the knees. Inhale. As you exhale, move one knee down towards the opposite ankle. Inhale and return to the start position. Try and keep the hips in contact with the floor throughout.

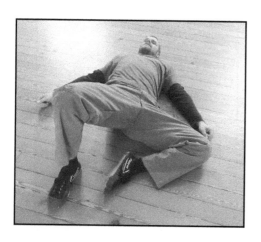

Repeat the last exercise, but this time the knee goes down to the outside.

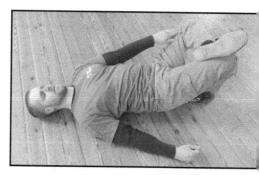

Place the feet flat on the floor, knees raised. Now take one ankle and place it on the opposite knee. Inhale. As you exhale, slowly push the knee away from you. Inhale and release the pressure.

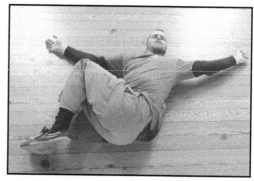

Bring the knees up a little higher, so that the feet are off the ground. Take the arms out to the sides. Inhale. As you exhale, take both knees across to the side and down. Inhale and return to the start position.

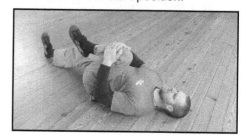

Lay back and raise one leg. Grasp the knee with both hands. Inhale. Exhale as you pull the knee up towards the chest. Make sure you keep the direction of the pull straight, do not pull out to the side.

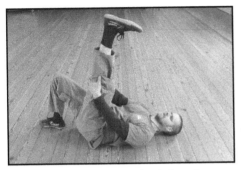

Lift the leg up and place both hands behind the knee. Inhale. Exhale as you straighten the leg and pull the knee towards the chest.

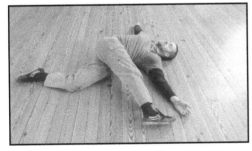

Lay back, with arms out to the sides. Inhale. As you exhale, take one foot towards the opposite hand. If you can reach far enough, you can grab the toes to hold the leg in place. Try and keep the shoulders in contact with the floor throughout.

Sit up with your legs stretched out in front of you. Inhale. Exhale as you lean forward to touch your toes. Try and keep the back straight, do not slouch. If you cannot reach the toes at first, just go as far as you can. If you can reach the toes, you can also pull them back to increase the stretch.

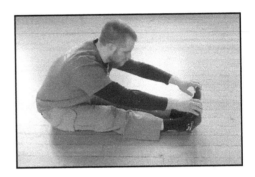

Sit upright and bring both legs out at an angle. Inhale. Exhale and take your hands out to rest on the shins. Keep the back straight. From the same start position, exhale as you lean forward. Try and place the palms flat on the floor. It is important again to keep the back straight. Slouching means the body gets lower, but you are not stretching so much!

Staying upright, grab the feet and pull them in together. If you can, bring the feet sole to sole. Inhale. As you exhale, lean forward and

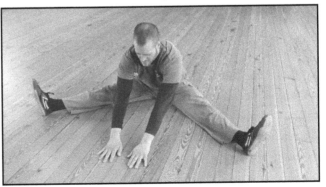

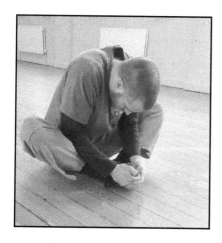

at the same time try and push the knees down. Inhale and return to upright position.

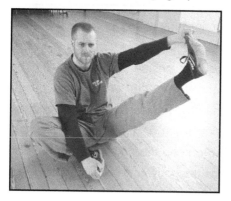

From the last position, grab the feet separately. Inhale. As you exhale, straighten one leg out, keeping a firm grasp of the toes. Inhale and return to the start position.

Stretch one leg out in front and fold the other back. You can use the hands to support your weight. Inhale. Exhale and lean the body forward, you can reach for the toes as before. Once again, be sure not to

slouch. An alternative is to have the rear leg bent forward, so the sole of the foot is against the inner thigh of the lead leg.

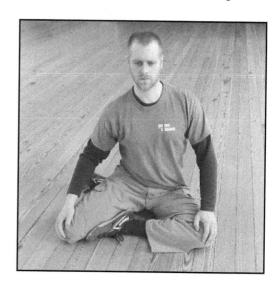

From the above position, bend the lead leg so that the sole of the foot rests against the rear thigh. This is a very good resting position and, like the Cossack Squat, you should try spending some time in it each day. Be sure to maintain a straight spine. You can apply a little pressure to the lead knee if it is lifting, but be gentle and work to relax the inner thigh muscles.

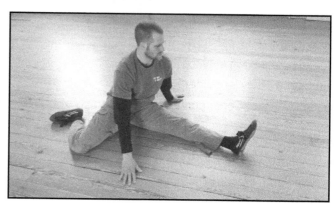

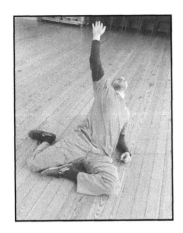

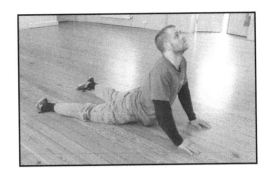

To stretch from this position, inhale. Then exhale as you raise the arm and lean back. You can support the body weight on your elbow as shown. Inhale and return to upright position. You can try the same thing

down towards the floor. Again we can follow the three move one static method, or whichever way suits best. Lay on your front with palms on the floor. Exhale. Inhale and raise the upper body as high as you can. Keep the hips flat and the lower back as relaxed as you can. Exhale and lower down.

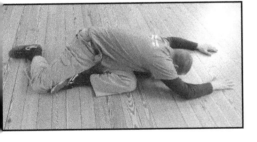

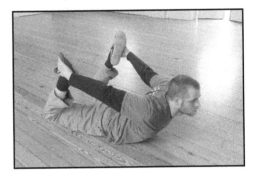

but leaning in different directions. Here, you can see how to bring the palms to the floor to get a good stretch for hips and lower back.

Our last few stretches work into the back - so again, take care if you have any issues, or check with your doctor before trying them. Whenever we arch the back this way, it is advisable to follow up by arching it forward. So after each of the exercises, get into a kneeling position and take your head

If you can, from the last position grab hold of your ankles. Exhale. Inhale and lift, exhale and down. This is a little more challenging, so take it easy!

So there is a selection of stretching exercises that will give you a good start. . Remember, it is all about relaxation, not forcing yourself into painful positions. Don't rush and, if running through them as a routine, do a little joint rotation and breathing before and after.

CHAPTER EIGHT
THE STICK

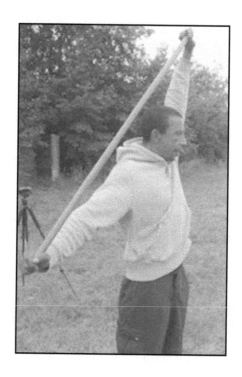

The stick is the single most useful object we can use in our training, particularly as we age. There is almost always some type of stick to hand, and, of course, some people use a walking stick regularly. What better item, then, to incorporate into our methods?

We use a stick for stretching, mobility, strength, balance and many other things. We will look at as many of those exercises as we can in this chapter, as you will likely find that stick work will form the core of your training.

First, what type of stick are we talking about? Well, we work with four sizes:

Small - a pencil, pen or similar

Short - around a foot or so in length

Medium - three or four feet in length, a walking stick, a broomstick or similar

Long - up to six feet or so in length, what in martial arts would be called a staff. A curtain pole or similar will do.

Whatever length of stick we should be sure it is suitable for use. The weight should be comfortable and the girth fit easily into the hand. The stick should be strong enough for purpose, especially for weight bearing exercises. We shall not be doing those so much in this book, but they are detailed in some of our other books should you wish to try them.

The next thing to consider is space and safety. Make sure you have enough room around you - even if doing quite small moves, it is easy to turn round and knock a vase off the shelf. If you are working in a group be sure to have enough space between people. Also check above - sticks are great at going through ceiling tiles!

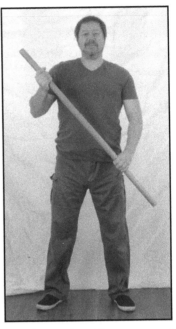

The first thing to do with any new object that we are using is to get a feel for it. So whichever type of stick it is, take a little time to hold it, move it around in the grip, get used to the weight and balance. For the most part we use the medium stick for training but you can experiment as you see fit. Naturally, our Four Pillars should be present throughout all of the following and, again, take it as read that we work both sides equally. We will start with some work on the hand, developing mobility and grip and the first exercises use a pen or pencil before moving up in size!

HAND TRAINING

These exercises can be done singly with each hand, or both hands at the same time. A few work both hands together, such as our first exercise.

Warm the hands up by placing a pencil between the palms and rubbing - as though you are starting a fire!

Place the pencil on a desk. Pick it up with the thumb and index fingertips. Put it down, then repeat with all the other fingers and thumb tip.

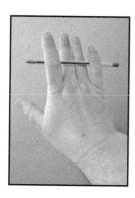

Place the pencil across the back of the two middle fingers as shown. Close and open the fingers, each time you open press the pencil.

Next place the tips of each hand at the end of the pencil and lift and put down. Again, cycle through each finger and thumb tip.

Place a pencil between the bottom joint of the little and fourth finger. Squeeze the pencil as hard as you can for a few seconds. Next, move the pencil up to the middle joint and squeeze again. Finally, move the pencil up to the tip of the little finger and squeeze again. We basically

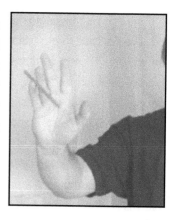

repeat this step with the pencil between each finger - so four times in all per hand. The trick is that you try and move the pencil from joint to joint or finger to finger without using your other hand! In other words, you have to kind of wiggle your fingers to move the pencil. This is a great drill not only for finger strength but also mobility.

Next, try moving the pencil continuously between the fingers, much in the same way a magician does with a coin. Use the tip of the thumb and index finger to swing the pencil round and go back again.

We will now move up to either the small or medium stick. Hold stick between the finger tips and walk the fingers up and down it (insy- winsy spider!).

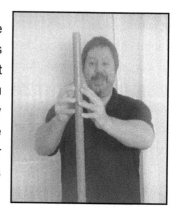

Next, work the same, but this time using just one hand. You can also try holding the stick in one or two hands horizontal too.

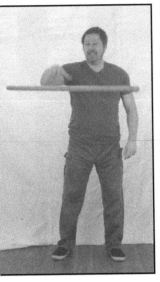

Hold the stick parallel to the floor. Drop and catch. Inhale as you lift, exhale as you drop. Each time you also move the hand a little along the stick. Start in the middle, work to one end, then back along to the other. Remember to keep the stick level.

Hold the stick in the middle with both hands. Turn the wrists up and down, as though working the throttle on a motorbike. Repeat with the hands in different positions, such as shoulder width apart and at the ends of the stick.

Hold the stick in the middle with one hand.

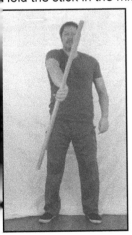

Twist the wrists so you are twirling the stick side to side. Start with quite small movements, g r a d u a l l y increasing. When ready, try and change hands without stopping the movement.

Hold the stick by one end at shoulder height. Allow the stick to drop, then circle it round to the start point again. At first, you can open the fingers, but try also to work it with closed fingers. Stop and reverse the direction.

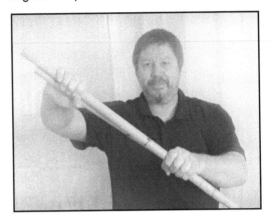

Get two sticks and twist them together, like trying to wring out a wet towel. Work the hands in different grips and positions.

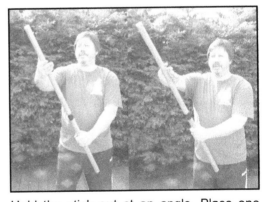

Hold the stick out at an angle. Place one hand on the outside edge and pull the stick towards you. Resist with the lower hand. Then place the resisting hand on the inside and push the stick away, again applying resistance with the lower hand.

ARMS AND SHOULDERS

Place the stick between the palms and, keeping the hands close to the body, rub

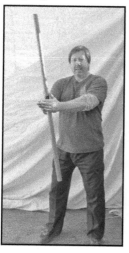

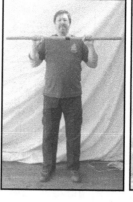

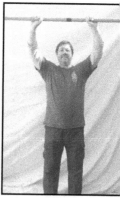

the palms together. Next extend the hands out a little further and repeat the same movement from the elbows. Finally, stretch the arms out full and repeat the movement from the shoulders.

waist. Lift to the chin and down.

Hold the stick palms up at the chest. Move the stick up and down. Keep the shoulders relaxed.

You can practice this next set of movements slowly, with a little selective tension, or relaxed and quickly to warm up the muscles. Either way, keep the breathing smooth.

Hold the stick in a palms up grip at the waist. Inhale as you lift the stick to the chin, exhale as it returns down.

Hold the stick in a palm down grip at the

Next we start making circles. Hold the stick out front, level to the floor. Make a large circle with the stick, both forward and back, keeping the shoulders relaxed. Try different grips and different hand positions.

Repeat the same movement but his time keep the stick in pace and circle the shoulders forward and back.

From waist height, circle the stick out to the side, up above the head, then back down.

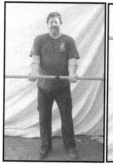
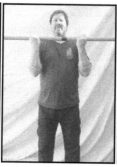
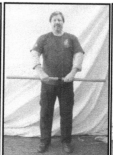
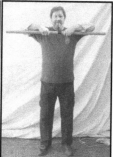

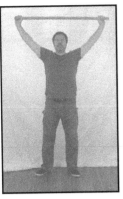
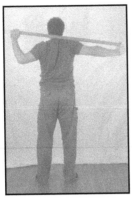
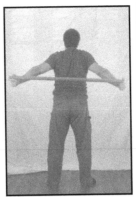
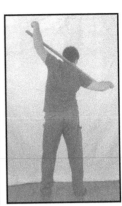

Alternate directions. Gradually bring the stick to behind the head. Hold it in place for a few seconds. Then work to bring the stick down behind the shoulders. See if you can work it all the way down to your waist at the back. You may find using a long stick more comfortable for this.

Place the stick across the shoulders. If you can, hang the elbows over the stick. If not, just hold the stick. Take care not to put pressure onto the neck. Begin making figure 8 movements, forward and backward.

TORSO

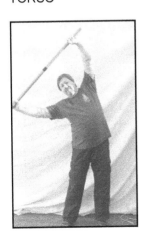

Lift the stick above the head, inhale. Exhale and bend to the right. Inhale to above the head, then exhale and bend to the left. From the same position, repeat

but this time turn the waist to the right and left.

From the same position, inhale, then exhale and bend forwards. Inhale and come back up. If your back is okay, you can lean back too on the inhale.

Hold the stick behind you. Inhale. Exhale and bend forward, lifting the stick as high as you can.

Hold the stick like a canoe paddle. Now begin a figure 8, nice and smooth.

With the stick held across the body, twist the waist side to side. Then add in figure 8 movements.

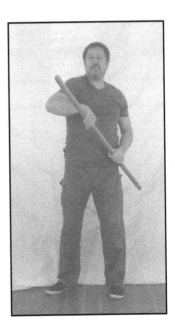

77

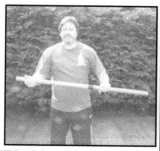
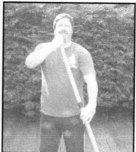
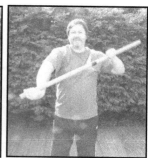

STRETCHES

Hold the stick at waist height left palm down, right palm up. Bring the right hand up towards your face, rotating the stick until it is above the right wrist. Pull down a little with the left hand for the stretch.

From the same start position, push with the left hand out to the right, allowing the shoulder to open. Keep the hips square and breath, let the muscles relax. Hold for a while, then repeat on the other side. Repeat but this time, pushing the stick backwards. Again, keep the hips square.

Drop the stick over the shoulder and grab it with the lower hand. Pull down gently as you exhale.

Hold the stick at one end and cup the other end with your palm. Push up with the lower hand as far as you can to stretch your sides.

Place one end of the stick on the ground, with both hands at the top end. Step back and bring the feet out little wider. Using the stick for support, lean forward. Be very sure to keep the lower back straight. Push the hips back a little. Hold while breathing. To raise up, bend the knees, push your hips forward and lead with the head. Be sure to straighten slowly.

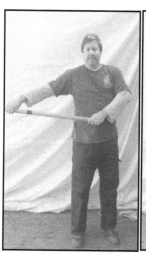
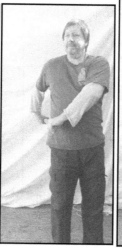
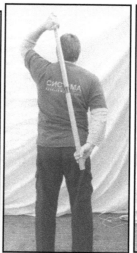
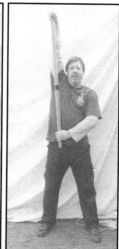

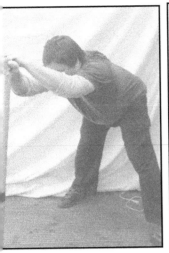
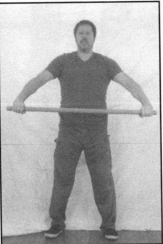
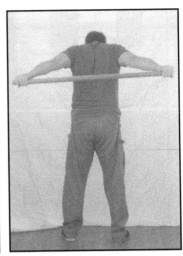

STRENGTH

Hold the stick at waist height. Apply selective tension in the forearms and push inwards. Maintaining the tension and very slowly lift the stick above your head while burst breathing. Relax at the top, then re-apply the tension and slowly lower to the waist.

Repeat, but this time pulling the hands outward. After that, repeat both methods out with the stick held behind you. Keep the tension in the forearms only, be sure to relax the chest and shoulders. You can vary the degree of tension to suit.

Hold the stick in one hand so that the other end is touching the floor. Working just from the wrist, slowly lift the stick to upright position, then back down again.

Place the stick across your back supported by the elbows - you need a stronger stick for this one. Apply tension in the arms, as though you are trying to break the stick

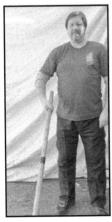
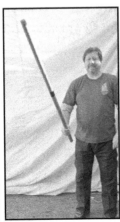
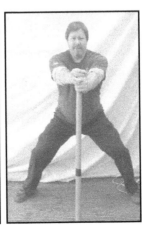
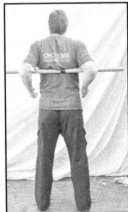

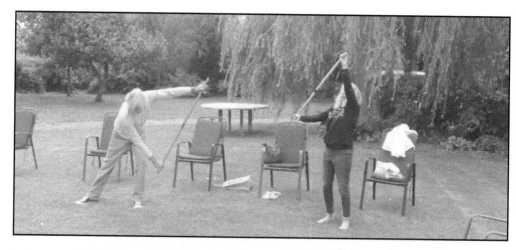

across your back. Remember to breathe. You can repeat with the stick held across the chest.

Place the end of the stick on the floor, with both hands on the top end. Go into squat position and, with selective tension, push down into the ground. Again, be sure you have a sturdy enough stick! Repeat with the stick held behind you.

GENERAL STICK WORK

There are many more stick exercises but the above will give you a good start. Once you are used to handling the stick, start to work more freestyle movement. Begin a movement pattern, say a one handed figure 8, then flow into another direction or pattern. If you have space, move around. Swing the stick with one or both hands, let it find its own momentum and move with it. Keep your posture, keep the breath working. Imagine the stick is a spear or a sword - sound effects are optional!

You can also try incorporating the stick into other exercises. Practice squats with the stick over your shoulders, for example. Or try ground movement while holding the stick. Again, be creative in your work.

STRETCH BANDS

We will finish this chapter with another piece of kit that is ideal for our purposes - stretch bands. A stretch band is basically a large rubber band that we can use to work our muscles without applying load to the joints. They are readily available and have the advantage of coming in different strengths, from light to XX heavy. This means we can select exactly the level of resistance to suit. Bands come in two sizes, the small ones are a foot or so long, the large ones about three times that.

Stretch band exercises are pretty straightforward. You exert force from one or both ends. Let's run through some simple examples, just to show how they work.

place and push the other end out with the palm.

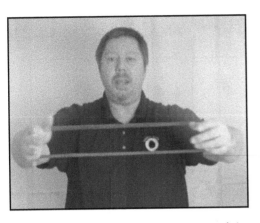

Loop the small band over your wrists. Inhale and stretch out to the sides. Allow the chest to open. Exhale and relax.

Think back to some of the stick exercises and work the same with the bands. From waist height, stretch the band then, maintaining tension, slowly raise the arms above the head. Repeat to the back.

You can also work with one end fixed. Hold on end at waist height, grab the band with the opposite fist and pull the hand up to work the upper arm.

The longer bands gives a few more options. For a wider stretch, grab each end and repeat the first exercise. Or fix one end in

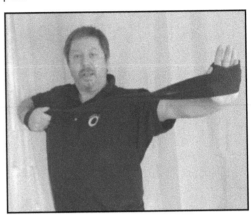

Another option is to stand on the long band, hold the upper part, then stretch up towards the chin. You can do this palms up and palms down.

You can use the bands on the legs too. Lay on the floor, place the short bands around the knees and open out to the sides, for example. Looking back at the leg stretches will give you some good ideas.

The good thing with the band is that you can control the amount of resistance and force and you aren't loading the joints. But always remember to breathe and exercise selective tension. Also be aware that if you let one end go the band can snap back!

Overleaf are two sets of exercises, standing/floor and seated. Once you have the idea, it is easy to make your own exercises too.

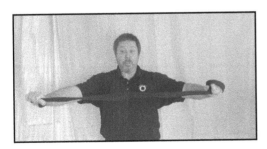

STRETCH BAND STANDING

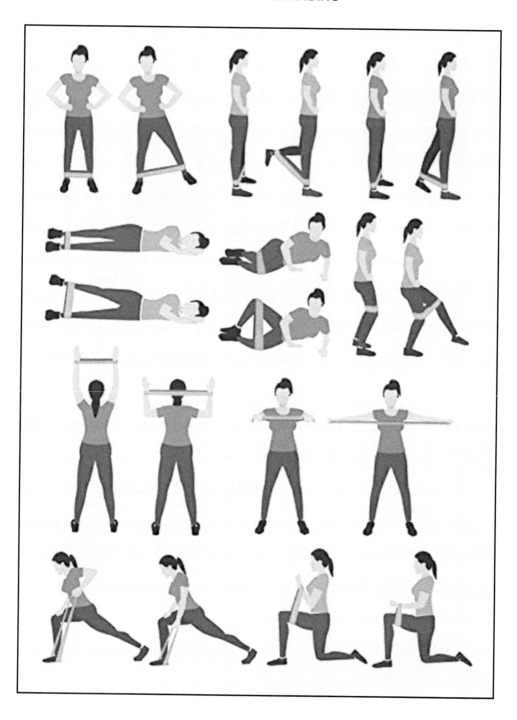

STRETCH BAND SEATED

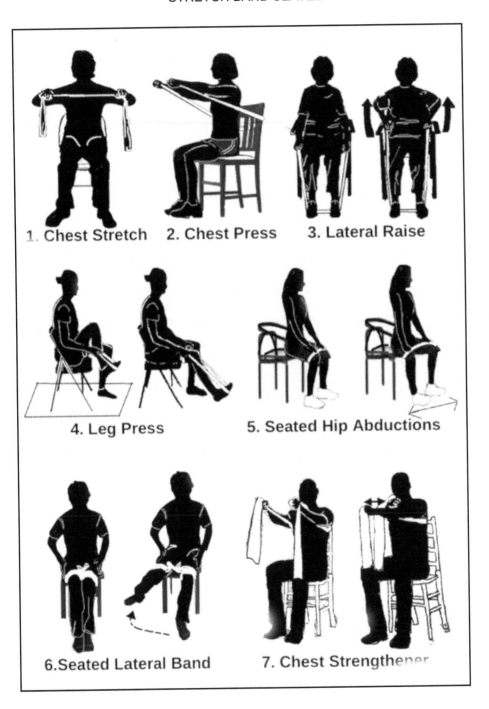

1. Chest Stretch   2. Chest Press   3. Lateral Raise

4. Leg Press   5. Seated Hip Abductions

6. Seated Lateral Band   7. Chest Strengthener

CHAPTER NINE
BALANCE AND FALLING

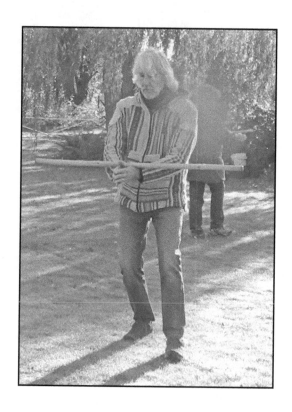

Worsening balance and the consequent falling are a major concern in seniors. In the UK, around a third of people over 60 and around a half of people over 80 fall at least once a year. Factors such as poor eyesight or hearing, lack of mobility, tension-created fear are some factors, along with the environment (rugs, ice, etc.)

I've always taught falling as an integral part of self-defence. Indeed, after breathing it is a foundation of our training, whatever a person's age. I doubt there is a person on the planet who has not fallen over at some time - whether through a broken paving slab, snow, age or alcohol! But, of course, if a person is already a little frail of has some condition, we must approach our falling work in a very steady and methodical manner.

Balance is one of our "extra" senses on top of the usual five. Our sense of balance involves eyes, ears, and also our body's natural sense of where it is in relation to itself - what is known as proprioception, Balance also involves our support structure - the joints, ligaments and stabiliser muscles that hold them in place. So any work on balance will also work these key features. Of course balance also relies heavily on posture - poor posture will not help balance! So by working on posture we are already improving our odds of staying upright.

The sequence we will follow here should allow people of almost any age or condition to develop some measure of balance improvement, falling skills and, equally important, the ability to get back up again. A few years back an elderly neighbour would frequently fall and remain "stuck" on the ground literally frozen with tension. This not only made him very heavy to lift, it also increased his risk of injury. Eventually I'm pleased to say he agreed to move into sheltered accommodation where he had help on hand 24/7.

We will start with some methods of improving balance, then next work to getting down onto the floor. From there, we will look at some suitable ground mobility exercises. After that, we will explore different ways of getting back up again, then finish the chapter by running through a sequence of falling exercises, literally from the ground up.

When teaching older people I've often found strong resistance to any kind of falling work. It provokes a lot of fear, people perhaps have visions of being asked to break fall or dive headfirst into the ground. That is not the approach we take and I would counsel that falling work is absolutely vital to learn as we age. Just take things easy, work up from the ground to whatever your limits are. You will at least gain experience in learning how to control the impact of a fall and so remove much of the fear and tension associated with it. The more afraid you are of falling, the more likely you are to fall, it is a self-fulfilling prophecy!

Find a safe and comfortable surface to work on too. For the floor work have something soft underneath and for all the work be sure there are no edges or corners near-by. Also be sure to have some support to hand - a chair, a stick or similar.

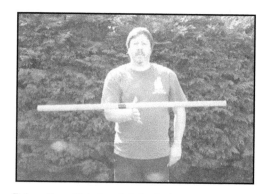

EXTERNAL BALANCE

We will begin with balancing objects outside of our body. We do this unconsciously every time we pick something up, we (hopefully) align it with our own centre of balance. However doing this in a more mindful way is a great way of both getting us into balance training and also fine-tuning our posture.

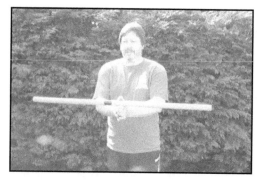

Grab a medium stick. Bring your palms together and balance the stick across your fingers. Find the stick's balance point and let it rest. If your posture is good this should be quite easy. Now, raise up one shoulder or tilt your hips and see what happens to the stick - it shifts, right? So we use the stick as an "antennae" in much the same way we did in the chapter on posture.

Bring the stick back into balance and stand for a minute or so. Check for tension, keep the breathing smooth. Now remove one hand, so that the stick is balanced on a single finger. Use the thumb to steady it if needed. Relax, breathe. Notice how any small movements in the body are amplified in the stick. After a time, switch hands.

Next, try balancing the stick end in the palm of the hand. More of a challenge, as the contact area is small and the whole weight of the stick is vertical rather than horizontal. Try not to "chase" the stick too much as it moves. Remember any move you make will be amplified. Instead, move gently under the stick to regain balance. This is a very important

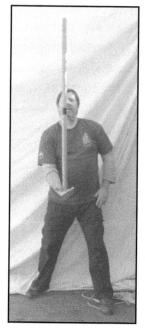

principle later on when we come to falling, so it is good to learn it here first. If you have space you might also take a small step or two in order to follow the stick.

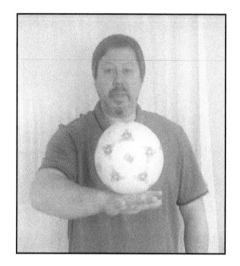

One more exercise for the hands. This time we use a ball - a small football or similar. Place the ball in the palm of the hand and balance it. This should be easy, the ball will sit in the curve of the palm, we have a lot of contact. Also, our palms are full of sensors, we are used to handling things and performing complex tasks with them.

For the next level, balance the ball on the back of the hand. Smaller contact area, convex shape and less sensors. As with the stick, try and use small, smooth movements to adjust your position under the ball, again this is great for developing tactile sensitivity and body awareness.

So, that is the hands, how about using other parts of the body? The head is a great

one, I'm sure some of you will have had to balance a book on your head at some time to learn how to "walk properly!" We used to do it in Tai Chi, running though the form with a book in place and I know dancers and others will have done the same. So let's start with a book. Get something suitable and place it on your head. Remember our earlier posture checks. If everything is aligned, this should not be too difficult. Breathe, relax.

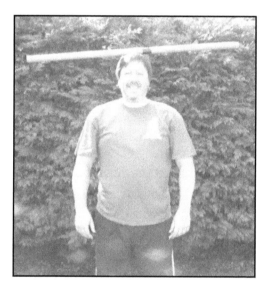

Try the same thing with other objects - the stick, for example. The ball may be too much unless your head is a bit flat or you have a big hair-do!

INTERNAL BALANCE

Let's now look at the actual balance of the body. When we are standing upright in our "at rest" position, our centre of balance is generally in the lower abdomen, just below the navel. In Eastern martial arts and disciplines, this is a focal point of training - as well as the balance centre, it is also said to be the main energy point of the body. Most work in those, consequently, is about sinking down into the legs and moving the body from the central point.

This is fine though, if not careful, it can bring a lot of pressure into the lower body, particularly the knees. It also suits an environment where you can "press" the foot down into the floor. However, for other types of surface, for people who are tall or for anyone whose hips are a little stiff, this can be an uncomfortable method.

In Systema we have a concept known as the Pendulum. Think back to our posture and walking work. The head is suspended from above. The shoulders are back a little, the chest slightly raised. The upper body lifts, allowing the spine to lengthen and the abdomen to open. The centre of balance here is more in the chest than in the belly. The hips should be free to move 360, swinging like a pendulum. The footwork will now be agile and light - something like a ballroom dancer rather than a karate expert.

With this in mind, we start by exploring the current limits of our balance. Stand upright in a neutral position. Rock the weight forward into the balls of the feet. Feel the point at which you lose balance - you can take a step or two to restore it. Repeat this a few times.

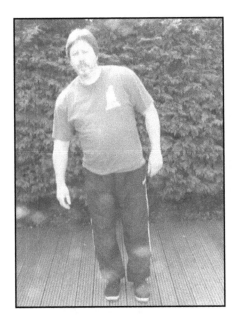

Next, move forward to the point where you are just keeping balance. Burst breath. Try and relax. You may feel the muscles in the lower leg and ankle firing in. That is good, this is one way of strengthening those important support structures. Hold for a minute or two.

Relax, and repeat the same drill to the back. Take the weight into the heels until you have to step backwards a few times. Then go to the boundary line again and hold. Try and pinpoint any tension in the body. Feel where the fear lives and work to disperse it with breathing.

Now work also to the left, then the right, taking the weight into the sides of the feet. Stumble a few times, then hold. This gives us an idea of our "zone of balance" from a normal position. Of course, our centre or zone will change according to the situation -

if our posture is twisted, or if we are carrying something heavy, for example. But let's stick with our "zone". Now circle your weight around the outside of the feet, working along the line of that zone. Perhaps like me you are old enough to remember Weebles! That's the movement we are looking for - if not, look it up. Or imagine you are on the deck of ship in a rough sea! Circle round in each direction, keep the breathing working. Test the limits of your balance, if you feel safe enough to do so.

Having established that, let's work some static balance drills. Stand as before and raise one foot off the ground - it need only be a couple of inches. Stand tall and breathe. Again, note where any tension develops. Allow your body to relax into your support structure The head lifts you up, the hips relax and rest on the supporting leg. Try to keep the hands down at the sides, avoid flapping them around if you can. Think stillness. Hold for a time, then switch legs.

Again, this drill will work to strengthen your support structure. It's something that can be done anywhere, anytime you are standing around for a bit. In fact, people who have to stand for long periods of time use this to rest one leg.

The next level is to raise one foot again and this time, close your eyes. This will have a major impact on your balance so make sure you are in a safe environment.

We are told that a person requires at least two of the following three senses to maintain balance while standing: proprioception; vestibular function (the ability to know one's head position in space); and vision (which can be used to monitor and adjust for changes in body position). If we take away the sight we have to rely on, and so hopefully improve, the other two. The medical procedure for this is know as the *Romberg Test.*

This is important because as we age, or even before, our eyesight can deteriorate, thus contributing to worsening balance. We can mitigate this to some extent by practicing

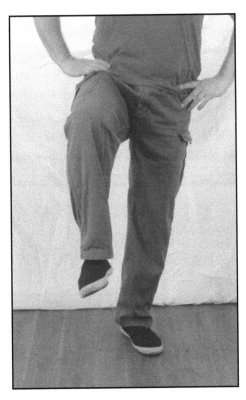

eyes closed static balance.

One thing you will find useful in this exercise is the breath - use short breaths to keep the body relaxed and to keep the mind centred. Allow everything to relax, again try not to snatch the air for support.

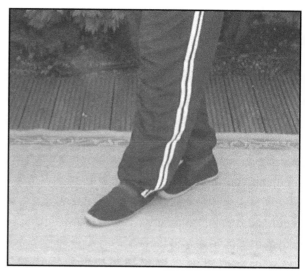

If you want to go the next level of challenge. Stand with feet together and eyes open. This time, lift the heel up and stand on your toes. This gives less surface area of support and also makes our base of support more precarious. Try this on both feet and one foot.

good posture will alleviate this and our earlier walking method helps do not only this but also minimises wear on the joints. So let's try a walking drill.

The pinnacle of balance drills is to stand on tip-toe with eyes closed - both and one foot as before! Now this is very challenging but if you can work through to this level you will develop exceptional balance!

So far, all of our balance exercises have been static. Naturally, when we move our balance will shift. To a large extent keeping

We call this the Tightrope Walk. Stand normally, we will be walking forward. Place the heel of one foot in front of the toes of the other, with contact. Imagine you are walking a long a tight rope. You can experiment with holding the arms out or keeping them at the sides.

Walk forward this way for as many steps as you like. To return, repeat the same step but going backwards. As always, breathe, relax. Keep an eye on the posture, try not to look down at the feet, this will tilt the head.

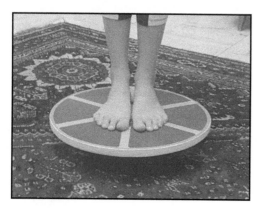

It is possible to buy "training tightropes" that sit a foot or so above the ground, or you can try walking on something narrow - but only if it is safe to do so and you are able to fall safely! The same thing goes for items like

obble boards or large gym balls. By all means try them it if you feel safe in doing o. At least with a wobble board you may e able to use something to give you upport if required.

Above all, train your balance every hance you get. When standing, lift one oot a little. This kind of regular work will ring the greatest benefits in terms of trengthening your support - and the better our support, the more confident and so nore relaxed you will feel.

Ve will finish this section by combining our xternal and internal balance. Take the tick, book or ball and start from those ame positions as before. Let's place the ook on the head, for example. Now take a few normal steps. Try doing some slow quats. Go up and down the stairs.

ry the horizontal stick balance drill again, his time combined with the Tightrope Walk. f you can do it with two hands, switch to ne!

As you can see, there are numerous oossibilities here to balance all sorts of objects as your go through your daily activities - it could even make hoovering un!

GOING TO GROUND

Let's now look at what happens when we lose balance. We start our falling training

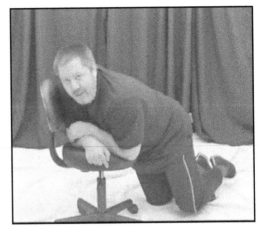

from the ground, which means first looking at some ways to get to the floor safely. It is best to think of this getting down and up work in terms of stages or levels.

Level 1 - Standing
Level 2 - Crouch or lean
Level 3 - Squatting
Level 4 - Kneeling
Level 5 - Sitting
Level 6 - Table Position
Level 7 - Prone on the floor

It is not necessary to go through all of the these levels, though even people falling fast go through most of them. How much time we spend in each depends largely on our experience and condition. A person used to this work can go from standing to squat to prone very quickly. For our purposes, we will spend a little time in each level, beginning with an assisted method.

Stand in front of a sturdy chair and hold the arms. Lean if you need to but try and

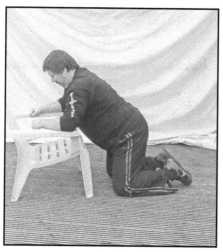

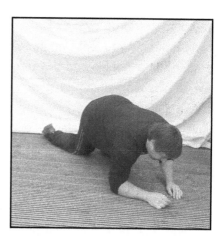

minimise the lean. Go into an assisted squat, then into a kneeling position. Use the chair to support the weight of the body.

Spend as much time as you like in each position, be sure you are stable before moving onto the next. From here, shuffle the knees back, and bring one hand and then the other to the floor, into the Table Position.

Alternatively, you could bend one elbow and bring the knee on the same side up towards it. Slowly lower and allow the body to roll to the side. Remember, we are trying to avoid impact with any bony part of the body, Keep the elbow tucked in, touch down with upper outer arm / shoulder and thigh. From here roll onto your back.

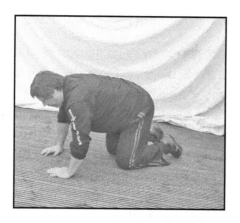

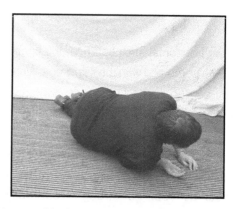

From this position you can slowly take your knees back then lower the body to the floor.

You could also use a low chair or footstool. Sit on the edge of it, supporting your weight through your arms. Slowly shuffle or slide forward and gradually lower yourself until you are sitting on the floor. From here, just lay back

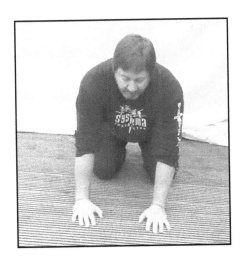

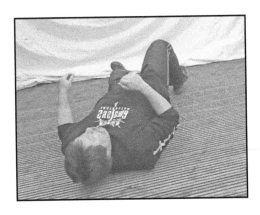

ON THE GROUND

If you are able to do movements like the Cossack Squat, it is quite a simple transition to the floor. Go into the Cossack Squat. Now lean forward an place your hands softly to the floor. Either walk your hands forward or slide your feet back until you are in Table Position. Roll onto the side, then the back as before.

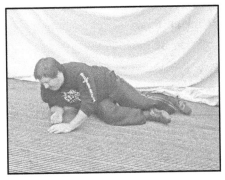

Generally we are looking to exhale as we change level down, to help the body relax. If you are working slowly, though, you could try burst breathing instead. Once you have the basic idea of levels, you can try your own variations depending on how comfortable and safe you feel.

Now we are on the floor, let's spend a little time getting comfortable there. Systema has a huge range of ground mobility drills, we will focus on a few here that best suit our purposes. Again, be sure to work on a soft surface, keep your movements slow and relaxed and remember to breathe.

While laying your back, run through some joint rotations. Work the shoulders, arms, hips and legs. Next, see if you can use these movements to shift yourself around a bit. For example, press the shoulder down to the floor and rotate it - you may find you are able to drag the body a little with this. Repeat on each side so you are "crawling" along the floor.

Try the same thing by pressing your heel into the ground and pulling the body towards the feet. Or push yourself around with your hands. See what sort of movement you can generate.

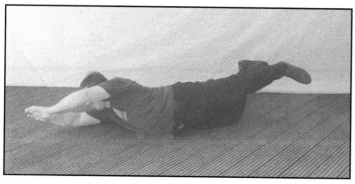

body forward, push and pull with the feet, etc.

To return to your back position, lift one arm or foot and take it across, again just let the rest of the body follow.

Next, we will roll onto our front. We do this by stretching out a foot or a hand and allowing the body to follow the movement. Imagine you are stretching out to grab something, for example. The fingers lead, the elbow and shoulder follow, then the chest and the rest of the body. Exhale as you roll.

Another method is what we call Threading. Lift one knee and push the other foot through the gap. As you do so, stretch the arms out, arch the lower back a little and allow the body to roll.

One more method of rolling from back to front is to bring the same side knee and elbow towards each other. As you do so, push the opposite shoulder forward and this should help you to roll, with the advantage of the move bringing you over onto your hands and knees.

Work again to see how much movement you have on your front. Use your hands / arms to pull the

So, the next thing is to get back up again! The main principle here, particularly if we are a little unsteady, is to bring as much support as we can under us before changing level.

GETTING UP

We start on our back. Let's assume we are a little frail and so are unable simply to sit up, then stand. First thing is to roll over onto our side and, from there, onto our front. As we come over onto our front, we are aiming to get on all fours, so the elbow to knee method may be most useful.

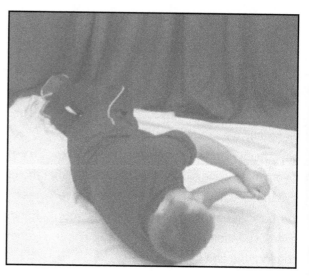

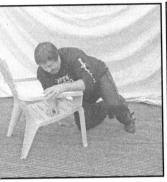 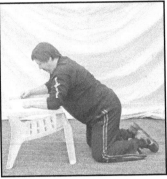 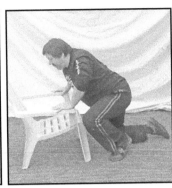

Once in our table position, we look for support. This may be a chair or anything similar that will support our weight without moving. Work to get as much upper body weight onto the object as you can. Next, bring the knees as close to under the hips as you can. Using the support, bring one knee up and place the foot on the ground. From here, slowly stand, keeping all your support under you. Don't lean or stretch out at all.

An option for standing up that we use a lot, is to work from a position we looked at in our stretching work. We first bring ourselves up to sitting position - either by a simple sit up or by kicking the legs out.

We place the sole of one foot on top of the other knee, forming a square shape with our legs. This is a good way to sit as we can easily move from this up, down, or sideways!

The next step is to move up onto the knees. Do this by raising the arms and expanding the chest - imagine this movement lifting your whole body up. Alternatively, you can use your hands on the floor for support.

From kneeling position, bring one foot round until its instep is pressed against the other knee. Now push down into that foot and allow the knee to open out and back. This will bring the body up without having to apply a lot of force with the leg muscles. The

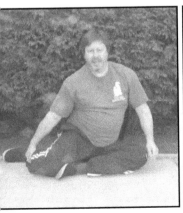 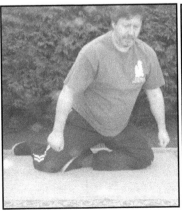 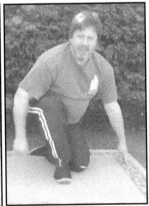

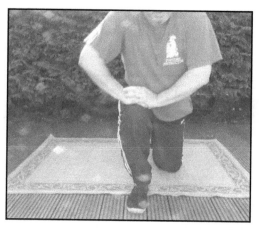

so we will learn some important principle: the first of which is to cover the head.

When we fall, we do not want he impact t send our head back into the ground Therefore, if you are falling backwards it i a good idea to cradle the back of the hea in one hand. It may not prevent impact bu will at least cushion it. Try and be aware when you go back, or keeping the hea forward a little and not letting it loll back.

rotation of the hip does most of the "heavy lifting" here rather than tense muscles. Remember to exhale as you lift.

You can also try bringing one foot out in front and using that knee as support. Place both hands on it and press down as you stand up.

FALLING FROM SITTING

Once we can get up and down without difficulty, we can being to work on actual falls. We start on the floor in a sitting position and will be falling back. In doing

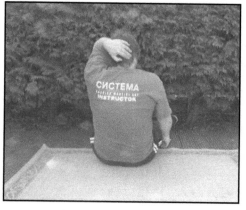

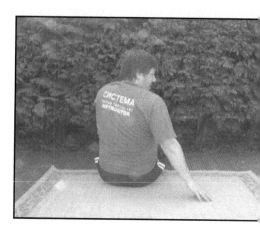

The second principle is the Sliding Hand When people fall, the natural response is to put the hands out, perhaps in an attempt to stop the fall. But the fall has already happened and all this usually achieves is damaging the wrist or elbow.

Experienced fallers can work without the hands, but if we do bring a hand out, here's what we should do. When the hand contacts the floor, do not lock it in place, but allow it to slide. This gives us a reference point to the floor, and helps best position the body for impact.

The third principle we have already touched on - hard floor, soft parts! We aim to keep bones and joints away from impact and instead land on our more cushiony bits. This usually mean tucking in the arms a little and rounding the body.

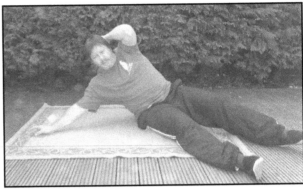

Let's revisit our earlier core exercise to help us put these principles into practice. Sit up straight. We are going to fall to our right first. So the left hand comes up to protect the back of the head. Take the right hand out to the side as you begin to fall in that direction. As the hand touches the floor, let it slide away from you. This should slow down your fall a little.

Turn into the fall so that you are coming down on the side of the body. Avoid landing directly on the spine. As the had slides, turn your palm up, rotating your arm. This should mean you effectively "slide" into the impact rather than crash down like a tree being felled. Exhale.

Sit up and try again. You can work the same side or alternate left and right. Practice this until you can do the movement smoothly and without any jarring impact.

FALLING FROM KNEES

Once we can fall from sitting, we go up to the next level, working from the knees. We can fall backwards again from here, but will also try falling forward. This leads us to another principles, the Folding Arm.

From a kneeling position, slowly fall forwards and allow one hand to touch the floor. You can practice sliding as before. Say it is the right hand, slide it across to your left which

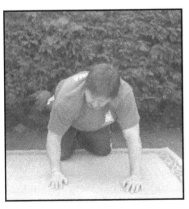
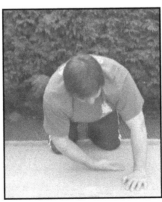
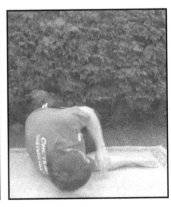

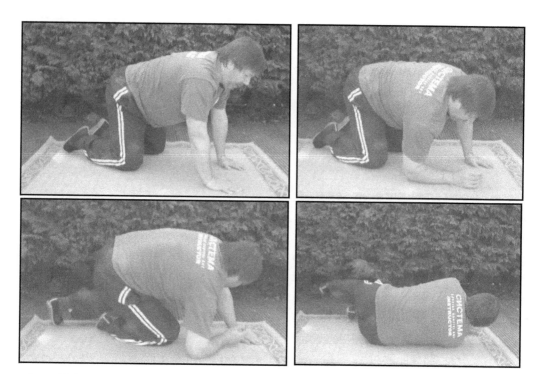

should bring your body down onto its side.

Another method is to fold the arm. Practice this from either the Table or push up position. Rotate the hand outwards, so the palm turns up. As you do this, lower the body, rotating the forearm until the weight is in the elbow. Then rotate the elbow in to bring the shoulder to the floor. Once the shoulder touches the floor, roll to the side, and from there onto your back.

Again, we are aiming for a controlled descent rather than a straight fall. Exhale! Practice from the static position then, when you are ready, from the fall.

From kneeling, allow the body to fall forward. Place one hand out, as it contacts

the ground, fold as above or slide as before. This should bring you smoothly down onto the shoulder. Don't worry if it's a bit bumpy at first, it takes a little practice.

FALLING FROM THE SQUAT

The next stage is to practice falling from the squat. We will fall backwards - remember the option of protecting the head with one hand, too.

From a squat, allow the body to fall back. As you go, turn ton one side a little so that you are not falling directly onto the back. Extend the hand on that side and allow it to touch the floor.

As it touches, slide, exhale and bring the

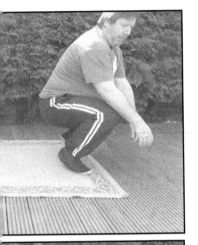

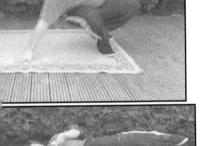

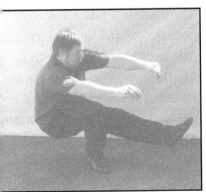

body down as slowly as you can, onto your side. From there, you can roll onto your back, onto your front, then work back up into a squat and repeat.

FALLING FROM STANDING

Going to ground from standing may seem daunting until you think back to our earlier "stages" list. If I can fall from sitting, all I have to do is sit, then fall! The aim then, is to control our descent down into one of our lower stages, then fall from there. Sounds easy!

To fall back then, we can work from standing into a squat and proceed as before. Simply stand, drop into the squat and fall.

We can also work by the "sitting" method. For this, we extend one leg out in front of us as we lower down. A little more leg stability is required for this one, in effect we are working a pistol squat, though not holding the position. So it might be good to practice this one with some support at first, from an object or other person.

Cup the head and take one foot out in front. Move down as though sitting on a chair and, once at the right height go into your rear fall.

How about falling from standing? We can work this in a couple of different ways. The first is to make ourselves fall by adjusting our stance. To do this, stand, then take one foot out as far as you can - and then a bit further! This will have the effect of giving you a slow fall, but you will also be lower to the ground.

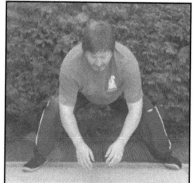

Of course, you can easily modify this to fall backwards or sideways too. This is a good method as, to some extent, it replicates a slip, where one foot slides out and away from us.

If you are feeling brave, you can practice it directly that way too, especially on a slippery surface. Allow one foot to slide away, or you might even use a tennis ball or similar to get the same effect - just remember to be careful.

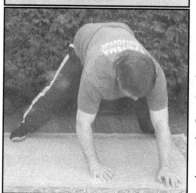

The other option for the forward fall is to bend at the waist, bringing the hands as close as you can to the floor before falling. Again, the lead hand should fold or slide and try to take the feet back as far as you can, this will create the space for you to fall into.

The final method, for now, is to fall to the side from standing. To work this, cross one foot back behind the other and allow the body to drop sideways.

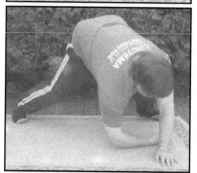

Try to go down rather than too far sideways, in effect going into a squat / sitting position. Extend the arm and allow it to slide out, bringing you down onto your side. From there you can roll onto your back as before.

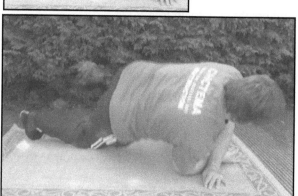

There is further falling work to be done in Systema, such as diving falls, rolls, twisting falls and so on. However, if you have never done any falling work before, the exercises here will give you a good method for any potential falls around the home, as well as serve as a good foundation

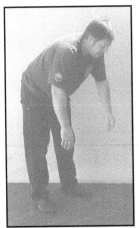

should you wish to explore the more advanced methods.

I would just stress again the importance of taking everything slowly and carefully and working in a safe environment. It might be good to only practice when another person is present, you can also help each other getting up and down. This in itself might be good preparation for if one of you does fall in the future.

A final thing to consider is if you have to help lift another person who has fallen. The first thing is that you should consider doing so only if it is safe and comfortable. If you are unable to lift them, call for help, do not put yourself at risk.

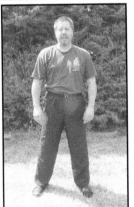

If you are able to help, then remember to observe all the usual rules of posture and use whatever support is required. Take it in stages, you don't have to lift them in one go. Think of yourself as the chair in the earlier exercise, you are a frame the person can use rather than a crane that is lifting them!

Never, never bend and try and lift the person in one go. If you have to lift, then squat, keep the back straight, place your hands under their arms and lift from your legs. Get the person into sitting position first, then work from there if need be.

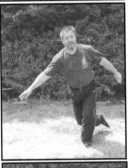

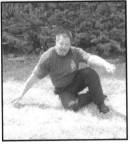

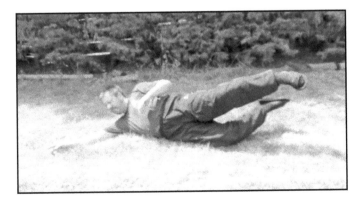

CHAPTER TEN
GENERAL HEALTH

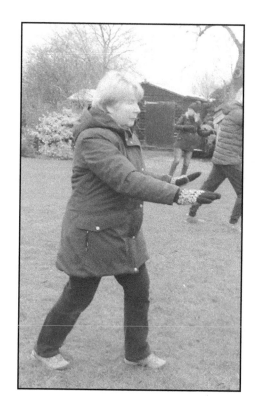

That covers the core aspects of Systema training for seniors. However, there are many types of other activity we can consider too, particularly rills to improve our general health and well-being.

We also need to consider other aspects of lifestyle that impact our health, as well as consider how to organise all this information into practical training routines. Let's start with some supplementary exercises.

COORDINATION

We know that older adults often experience a decline in motor coordination. Age related changes are caused by the loss of function to multiple areas of the brain. As we age, the neuromuscular communication in our body isn't as strong as it was earlier in life. A recent study found evidence that age-related changes in visual perception may also affect hand-eye coordination. The study showed that younger people interpret and react to near-body space in a different way than older adults.

Age isn't the only thing that can cause a decline in hand-eye coordination, however. Many neurological disorders can impact this function. Some of these disorders are more likely to emerge with age. Any movement we make requires communication from the brain. If these pathways are compromised, as they can be with disorders such as multiple sclerosis and ataxia, hand dexterity and responsiveness will decline.

Our exercises, then, have a strong mental as well as physical component. This means practicing activities that develop new neural pathways. Neural pathways are groups of nerve fibres which carry information between the various parts of the Central Nervous System. Think of it as the body's wiring! Any electrical appliance that has a loose connection will not function properly until the connection is fixed. Fortunately we can "fix" ourselves by developing new neural pathways.

We do this by practicing new behaviours - movements, learning things and so on. It has been shown that connecting new behaviour to as many areas of the brain as possible helps with this. In other words, tapping into all five senses creates a "stickiness" that helps form neural pathways.

Many of our Systema exercises work on cross-body communication - this improves the function of the nervous system and develops those new pathways. They can also help with balance and general coordination. As we have mentioned before, all of these areas are inter-linked, improving when usually helps one nor more others.

I bet most of you at some time have tried patting your head with one hand, whilst rubbing circles on your belly with the other!

This is a classic cross-body exercise involving left/right brain integration. So there is one that you already know, let's try something similar.

Clap your hands together in front of the face. One hand now touches your nose, the other touches its opposite shoulder. So, clap, right hand touches nose, left hand touches right shoulder. Clap and repeat on the opposite side.

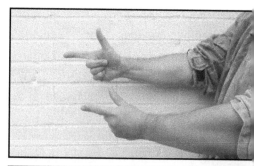

Here's another hand drill that is harder than it looks! Place both hands out in "pointing" position, finger out, thumb up. Retract the thumb on one hand, the finger on the other. The drill is to switch - so if it is left thumb up, right finger out, you have to switch to right thumb up, left finger out. You have to do both simultaneously. Give it a try!

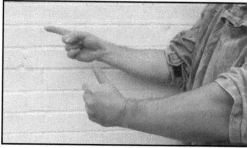

Next we move on to using the whole body. In fact we have already done one version of this exercise - our core movement where we raise opposite foot and hand. So feel free to re-visit that.

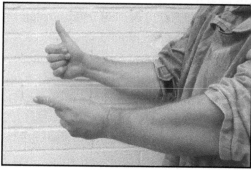

We will now describe the standing version, but if you find this hard , you can work the same movements sitting or even laying down.

Stand with feet shoulder width apart. If your balance is okay, lift the right knee up and place it down a few times. Then simultaneously lift the right knee and the left arm, and bring both down again. After that, repeat with the left knee and right arm a few times. Finally, alternate between the two, as though you are marching on the spot. Focus on synchronising the movement of the limbs - and don't forget to inhale / exhale!

After that, go back to your standing position. We will next work across the body's midline. Now, as you lift one knee bring the elbow of the opposite arm to meet it, as close as you

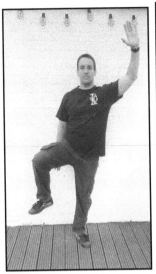 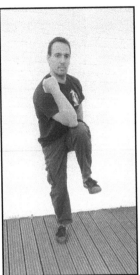

Imagine a large number on the floor, you have to walk its shape.

After that, combine both the arm movements and the walking. So as you walk the number three, you are also drawing it in the air.

Now go back to the start. Follow the same procedure as before but this time, you are drawing letters. It can be A,B,C etc or you can write out your name, for example. Run through with hands, feet and then walking.

can. Alternate as before with the focus on quality of movement.

I'm sure once you have the idea, you can see how easy it is to develop your own exercises. Even switching dominant hands can help - if you are right handed, try doing some things left handed, for example. We will finish with a set of exercises that involve letters and numbers.

Using one arm, draw out the numbers one to nine in the air in front of you. Repeat with the other arm. Finally, do the same with both arms.

Then follow the same procedure with each foot (seated if you balance is not good). For drawing with both feet you can sit down too!

The next stage is to "walk" the numbers.

The final stage is to try the walking but combining both drills. Walk out your chosen letters, while drawing the numbers with your arms and vice-versa. This takes some getting used to, so take your time!

As a parting thought on this topic, naturally any new activity that involves hand-eye coordination will help - some sports, juggling, playing a musical instrument, even some types of video game! The main point is that we are trying something new, giving ourselves a new challenge.

The same largely applies, of course, on a purely mental level. Studies of cognitive ageing find that the people who do more mentally stimulating activities have better thinking skills in older age. This can be as simple as doing things like crosswords, number puzzles, board games, memory games and so on.

Also look at working your basic observation skills. We cover a wide range of these in our *Systema Awareness* book but as a general guideline be observant when you are out and about. When walking, for example, shift your focus from things very close to you to things at far distance. Scan what is around you with all your senses. Take your time, don't rush and above all, as so few people do these days, keep your phone in your pocket! You will find yourself noticing things you never saw before. Of course, this is also a major component of our self defence training.

Other tips are watching films with the sound turned off (see how much of the story you can pick up visually), moving in low-light or even blindfold (in a safe environment, of course), sitting somewhere public where you can observe people (can you guess their occupation?) and giving yourself a running commentary as you are driving (junction twenty feet ahead, etc.)

EYE EXERCISES

We have mentioned vision in relation to balance and coordination. Eyesight is one area where most of us see a deterioration (speaking as someone who now needs glasses to read a newspaper!). There are some exercises we can do to assist and to strengthen eye function

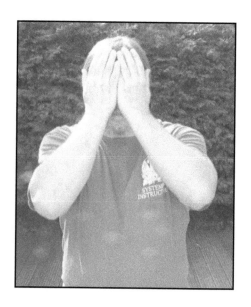

Sit in a comfortable position. Focus on your breathing, begin to slow it down. Let the body relax, particularly the head, neck and shoulders. Rub the palms briskly together until you develop some heat. Now place the palms over the eyes. You can experiment with keeping the eyes open or closed. Allow the heat to envelop the eye, particularly all the muscles around the eye socket. Hold for a couple of minutes.

Following this, rub the hands together again and begin to gently massage around the eyes. Do not press on the eye itself, but work into the sockets, under the eyebrow and down the sides of the nose. When finished, sit quietly for a few minutes with eyes closed.

Eye circles will help tone and stretch the eye muscles. Get into a comfortable position and keep your eyes open. Slowly move your eyes in a clockwise direction. Do this 20

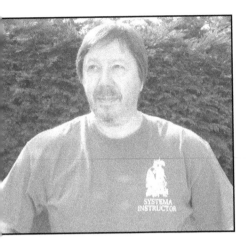

this position for 15 seconds. Do not blink. Slowly return your eyes to the original position. Close your eyes. Relax for 20 seconds. Open your eyes and look up between your eyebrows. Focus your eyes on this point for 20 seconds. Return your eyes to the original position. Quickly blink your eyes 10 times. Close your eyes. Relax for 20 seconds. Repeat this exercise three times throughout the day.

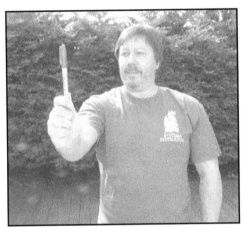

mes. Make as wide a circle as you are omfortable with. Relax for 10 seconds, nen repeat in a counterclockwise direction. Do this exercise three times daily. If having our eyes open for this exercise is too discomforting, close your eyes. You can also help your body wake from sleep by doing this exercise as soon as you awake.

Next, two focus exercises. Sit upright, hold a pen with your right hand, and straighten your right arm in front of your body. Keep he pen upright. Breathe regularly as you focus your eyes on the pen's tip. Focus for en seconds. Slowly bring the pen towards your nose by bending your arm. Keep ooking at the pen tip. Hold this position for five seconds. Slowly extend your arm again, all the time focusing your eyes on the pen tip. Hold the position for five seconds. Do not blink your eyes. Relax for ten seconds. Repeat three times.

Lower your eyes and gaze at the tip of your nose. Breathe as you regularly would. Hold

Contractions will strengthen and stretch weak eye muscles. Sit upright, palms on your lap, palms facing upward. Place your feet firmly on the floor. Tightly contract your eye muscles by closing and squeezing your eyes together. Hold this tension for four seconds. Open your eyes. Quickly blink your eyes 15 times. Relax for 5 seconds. Repeat this exercise five times throughout the day.

We can also strengthen our eye muscles with vertical movements. Sit upright and look up at the ceiling. Hold for five seconds. Return your eyes to the straight-ahead position. Relax for six seconds. Move your eyes to look down at the floor. Hold this position for five seconds. Return to the original position. Blink quickly 10 times. Relax your eyes for 20 seconds. Repeat this exercise four times.

Lastly, sit down, pick a point on the floor about three metres in front of you and focus on it. Trace an imaginary figure eight with your eyes. Keep tracing for 30 seconds, then switch directions.

Another thing to remember is that human eyes are not supposed to be glued to a single object for extended periods of time. If you are looking at a screen for a long time, practicing the 20-20-20 rule may help prevent digital eye strain. To implement this rule, every 20 minutes, look at something 20 feet away for 20 seconds.

MASSAGE

Massage is probably the oldest form of healing. It is such a natural thing - a parent will soothe their child through massage, we rub our temples when we have a headache and so on. Good massage brings benefits on many levels. It relaxes muscles, aids posture, and restores the skeletal system to its proper form. Massage can also stimulate blood circulation and the lymphatic system and aid with soft tissue damage.

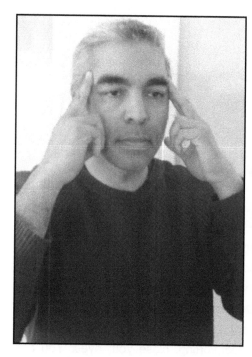

Systema employs many types of massage. For the purpose of this book we will show some self-massage techniques that are very simple and effective.

Sit down and run through a couple of minutes of Circular Breathing. Then rub your hands briskly together for a minute. Now, using the fingertips, start to gently press and massage around the eyes. Do not put too much pressure on the eyes themselves. Work under the eyebrow ridge, into the corners, and underneath the eyes. There are many small muscles in this area that hold a lot of tension, so take your time with this part of the massage.

Bring the fingers up to the temples. Press and make small circles, working into the muscle. Again, be sensitive to the amount of pressure you need - too little achieves nothing, too much may create more stress.

Work up onto the forehead, making small circles. Work along the scalp line and back out again, then a little lower down across the forehead itself.

Next, place the fingers in the corner of the eyes and work down the sides of the nose, applying light pressure. This will help with any sinus issues.

Rub out onto the cheeks and across the top lip. Sweep out to just in front of the ears and massage the jaw hinge. There is often a lot tension stored here.

Rub the palms briskly together again, then place over the ears. Feel the heat working into the muscles. Massage all around the ear, inside and out. Place fingers under the earlobes and work from here down under the jaw line to the point of the chin. Return to earlobes and repeat a couple more times.

Next, rub the hands together again, then"wash" the whole face with the palms.

Now we start to tap the scalp. Place the hands above the head and lightly tap with the fingertips. Start at the crown and work down and back. Then return to the crown and go down the sides. Finally, from the crown again, work forwards.

Link the fingers together and place the hands on the back of the head, so that the thumbs rest at the top of the neck. Applying pressure, run the thumbs down the large muscles at the back of the neck. Lift and repeat a few times.

Place your right hand on your left shoulder. You can support it at the elbow, if you like. Massage into the muscles of shoulder and neck with a "kneading" motion. Repeat on the right shoulder.

Vigorously rub the arms, chest and stomach with the palms. Rub the thighs, all around the knees and the calves in the same way. Have a little breathe and stretch, then get up and resume your day!

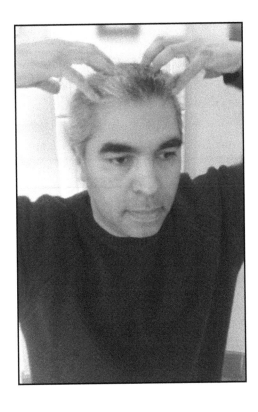

There are a few simple items we can use to help with massage, particularly trigger points. A hard rubber ball is great for working into tense muscles. Roll it on the floor with the sole of your foot, or sit and use it along the muscles of your calf and thigh. A larger ball can work the same for the back muscles. Simply place your weight on it and roll slightly.

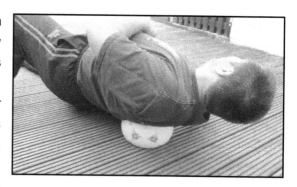

You can use a short stick to work into the long muscles in the body, particularly the legs and abdomen. Apply firm pressure as your brush the stick along the muscle length. This will also work nicely as a partner massage into the shoulders. Remember to avoid contact with the joints and bone.

Foam rollers are readily available and come in different sizes. Use a smaller one in the same way as the ball. Get a larger one to work your back. To use, lay across the roller and use your bodyweight to apply

moderate pressure to a specific muscle or muscle group. Next, roll slowly, no more than an inch per second. When you find areas that are tight, pause for several seconds and relax as much as possible. Remember your breathing! You should slowly start to feel the muscle releasing, and the pain lessen.

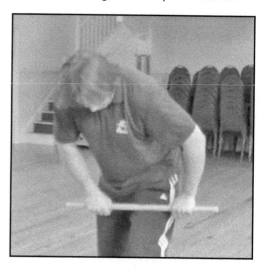

If a spot is too painful to apply direct pressure, shift the roller and apply pressure on the surrounding muscles. Work to relax the whole area, then go back to the original spot. You can also use the roller for the limbs, working on a hard surface.

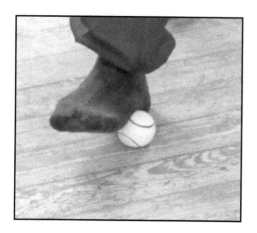

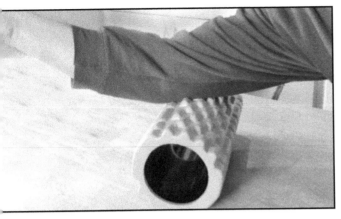

The first step is simply to splash cold water on your face first thing in the morning - we all know how that feels, right?

From there, when you have a shower, finish it by turning the water cold. You can try for maybe five seconds at first, then gradually increase

COLD WATER DOUSING

Another major Systema health practice involves cold water. This is something present in many cultures and health systems and ranges from splashing your face with cold water to breaking ice and jumping in the water! For this book we will give an introduction to the basic methods for you to try - again, under medical supervision if required.

So what does dousing do? In response to cold, the body shoots up its core temperature to over 40 degrees, which kills off most viruses and bacteria. It stimulates many of the body systems and will increase your resistance to cold. From an "energy" perspective, some claim it cleanses the energy field and helps us reconnect with the earth (hence being barefoot). Overall, it will wake you up and give you a warm glow and will also strengthen you psychologically in much the same way that fasting does.

the time. After a while, try the whole shower cold. Remember to burst breath and should you feel any dizziness or similar, exit the exercise.

The final stage is the full douse. Here we stand barefoot and pour one or two buckets of cold water over ourselves. Prepare your bucket before hand and it is good to let it stand for a while. If the weather is quite warm, you might want to add some ice to the bucket so the water really is cold! Stand in a

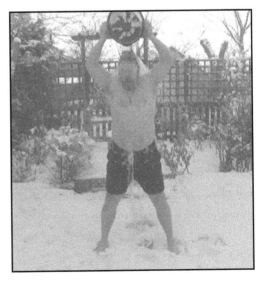

comfortable position and inhale. Raise the bucket and slowly and smoothly pour the water over the crown of your head, as you exhale. Following this, burst breath a little, especially if you are out in cold weather. It is good to do this practice on a regular basis, once or even twice a day if you have time.

It is best to start the full douse when the weather is quite warm, as this is a little more comfortable. But with regular practice you will be able to douse even in the coldest conditions. Just remember to burst breathe and wrap up warm quickly afterwards.

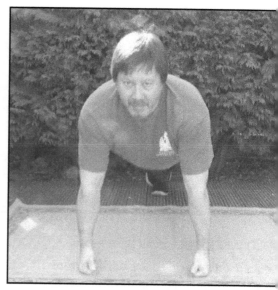

HOW TO TRAIN

Over the previous chapters we have covered scores of exercises, not mention all the variations that can be applied to most of them. This can all seem very daunting if you are not already training, or have not exercises for a while. So how do we start to organise this information into some type of regular routine? There are three things to consider: your current condition, your goals, and time / resources available.

Your current condition determines which type of exercises are available. If you have severe mobility issues, for example, then running and walking are probably off the cards. There are two ways around this - we do only the exercises we are able too, o we modify exercises so that we are able to do them.

Take our Joint Rotation work. Almost all o this can be done sitting or laying down. Ditto with stretching and some of the stick work In fact, you can also look at using the chai as part of the exercise. Grab the arm to help you twist the waist, for example.

If you are bed-bound or similar, then work any type of mobility you can, even if it is just wiggling your fingers. The breathing exercises are there, of course, but also consider visualisation. One of my students recently mentioned how, during a particular stressful time, she was running through the exercises in her mind. This is a surprisingly powerful practice, if nothing else it is good activity for the brain. There have also been studies done where people went into hospitals and performed Tai Chi and other exercises in front of bed-bound patients, with positive impact. Again, engaging even just the brain in some aspect of exercise has benefits.

Next, we consider our goals. To improve mobility? To feel fitter? Perhaps there is a specific event we are working towards. I know of a father who wanted to walk his daughter down the aisle, for example, certain exercises helped him achieve that. Or our goals may be more general - we just want to keep active and happy!

Either way, select which exercises will work best for you in attaining your goal. Don't be afraid to mix and match, or to take things from other sources - as long as they are safe. Don't be too rigid in your goals, and also consider that sometimes an activity has many other benefits beside the obvious.

I find that some younger people, for example, like to pursue strength above anything else. They do not understand yet that mobility is its own form of strength. In their eagerness they sometimes also train to injury, which becomes totally counter-productive.

Having established condition and goals, next look at your resources in terms of time, space and equipment. I have tried to keep to activities that require minimal equipment. I'm certainly no fan of expensive gym equipment and the various gimmicks available. As I hope I have shown, you can achieve a lot with just a broomstick! Of course, there is nothing to stop you investigating good methods such as kettle-bells and similar, as long as you get your information from a good source. When a new trend emerges, there are instructors who jump on the bandwagon and present material with little depth, so just be aware of that when looking at other methods.

In terms of space, you don't need a lot of room to do these exercises. I've stuck to solo work here as well, in order to minimise space and because you may not have a

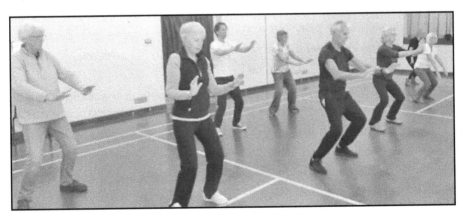

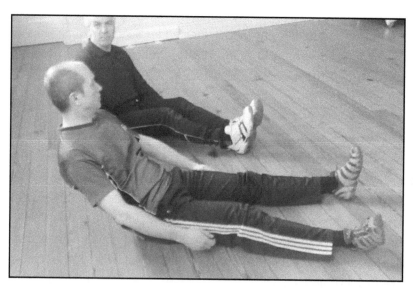

partner you can work with. Of course, Systema has numerous exercise drills for two or more people but it is best at first to get a good solo grounding.

If you have access to a local Systema class, then that solves a lot of problems! However, I would still not neglect solo training. If you can't find a Systema class, then consider things like pilates, swimming, any good movement and breathing type activity and so on. I would be wary of gyms that advertise "Exercise for Seniors." Some may be okay but my experience is that they give you the same as the "young person" class, just a bit slower. If there is no emphasis on posture or breathing, and everything is numbers based, I would go somewhere else.

The mention of numbers brings us to time and organising an actual session. At the

start, it is not a bad idea to give yourself a set number of reps. Let's say you have ten minutes available and want to loosen up a bit. Think along the lines of:

2 minutes breathing with selective tension

6 minutes joint rotation, eight reps of each movement

2 minutes do five reps of push ups, squats and sit ups, with recovery breath

I tend to start every session with some breathing and always make sure that my breathing and pulse are back to normal before I finish the session.

Using this method you might fit in a few ten minute sessions throughout the day. The morning can be for stretching, mid-day joint rotation, evening for core exercises. This is more my personal method these days. Rather than do one block of an hour's

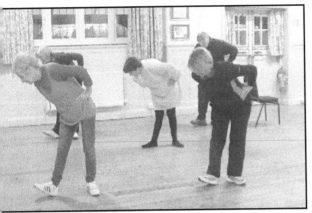

active, but with a focus and purpose.

Speaking of focus, you can practice any of the activities here in a mindful way - in that sense, you should always have an eye on posture, tension, etc. But it's also okay for some to have some music going or have the TV on. For some sessions I like listening to a podcast on the headphones. This also gives me a length for the session without having to check the clock. At other times, when doing more focused breath-work, for example, I prefer no distractions. Again, mix and match to suit your circumstances

Don't feel that every session has to leave you a sweating, panting wreck, either! There is nothing wrong with working cardio, which you can do with many of these drills. But our underlying focus is always on mobility and posture, developing our core, our balance, in short developing the key attributes that

aining, I do three or so blocks which fit in round my work and other activities. I then supplement this with a few bike rides a week to keep up my cardio - and to get out f the house in current lock down!

Another method is to assign different days o different things. Monday is stick day, Tuesday stretching, Wednesday floor work and so on. Or you might like to practice one particular skill, such as falling, over a period of a few weeks, or until you get it."

The main thing is that with the huge variety of activities available, you should never get bored. I remember hating gym back in my school days. Everything was rushed, it was the same session every time, the only point seemed to make you get out of breath. It was one thing that attracted me to martial arts - the prospect of being physically

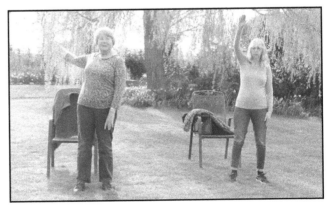

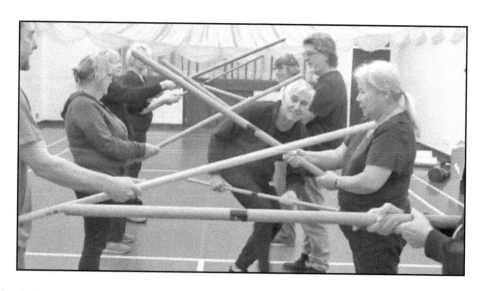

feed into our daily lives. I'm highly opposed to the kind of "fitness Olympics" currently out there. To me, fitness is not a race or a competition, any more than playing music is. That doesn't mean we become lazy and neglect our training but we should, by now, be beyond needing "special prizes" for our efforts.

In short, organise your training to suit your needs and circumstances. Once you have the basics, don't be afraid to experiment and adapt, creative thinking is a big part of the Systema approach. Check out all the resources available for further ideas, look at Youtube and similar, or where you can join a suitable class or on-line session.

TEACHING SENIORS

If you are an Instructor and have some seniors in your class, or perhaps want to start a senior specific class, what sort c things should you be watching out for?

Much of it depends, of course, on the condition of the people involved. We have some older gentlemen in our regula groups, a few of them are former Paras anc they like - they tend to be fitter than the younger guys! However, regardless of age we all pick up injuries or conditions that may limit our activities to some extent.

In this respect, our approach is nc different, then, from any other Systema class. We ask everyone to be open with any medical issues or conditions they may have and train with an eye to those, both in themselves and in their partners. Everyone works to the best of their capabilities.

Having said that, if the older people are experienced, I generally steer them more towards attribute development, mobility, posture and so on. Younger students I work more into fitness, strength development, more demanding mobility drills, etc. Now of course , there is considerable cross-over and one of the strengths of Systema is that everyone can be practicing the same drill with a slightly different emphasis according to their needs.

If you are running a specific senior class, then you can tailor things directly to the group. I started such a group about a year ago and one thing I learned very quickly was to stop thinking of the group as being "fragile!" Sure, I wouldn't have them doing dives over a chair, but, outside of that, the group does pretty much the same exercises as my "fighty" class.

One thing I found that the senior group really enjoys is some of the more "playful" aspects of group drills. Things like two rows holding out sticks and one person has to thread their way through them. The physical play element is something that tends to disappears in later life, so it's nice to watch people re-connect to it.

With a group of any age there is always a social element too, of course. So build in time for a little chat at the end - remember, your students may not get the chance to see other people face to face so much.

I also know of people who go into homes to run classes. In these cases, you may be working with people who have more restricted mobility. That's fine, as already mentioned, we can adapt almost all the work to sitting. One tip when working with seated people - sit down yourself to talk to them. Or, if you are close, kneel down to be on their level, don't loom over them.

If people are bed-ridden, than, again, sit beside them. A little contact may also be nice - hold their hand, for example. You can show them some breathing exercises, or perhaps some small movements.

Overall then, be patient, take your time in showing and explaining things and, above all, make the sessions as fun and laughter-filled as you can. It really is the best medicine.

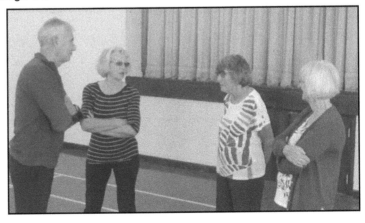

CHAPTER ELEVEN
LIFESTYLE

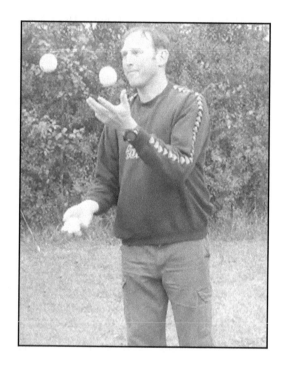

Obviously the type of life we lead has a huge impact on our health and ness. From diet to activity, or lack of activity, worries and stress, our relations with others and so on. Most of these are universal, and, for a comprehensive look stress management I would point you to my book *Don't Worry*, which details several methods fro stress management.

However, there are some areas which come with age, so let us discuss those. I think the two biggest issues that concern seniors are failing health and the lack of mobility it brings, and social isolation.

In terms of health, I hope that the methods in this book do something to restore or retard any physical issues that the reader may have. I also believe that good, regular activity of this nature will also do much to act as prevention rather than cure.

As well as the more physical activities, Systema has a number of supplementary health practices. We will details these briefly here, and encourage you to investigate them further should you require more information.

DIET

We are all aware of the importance of a good diet. In general, for me, that involves avoiding processed foods and using fresh ingredients as much as possible. This may involve a little more time in preparation and cooking but I think gives us a deeper connection, both with the process and also the people we are making food for.

If we live alone, it is easy to slip into the habit of cooking less, relying on ready meals, or even of not eating much at all. In that case, or if you live with a partner, I would suggest you set aside at least one time in the week for a "proper" sit down meal. It might be a three course dinner, it might be a cooked breakfast. But arrange the time and stick to it. Prepare and cook the meal yourself, lay the table, switch off the TV and phones. Spend a little time enjoying eating, whether alone or with others.

Another option, if you live alone, is to arrange a regular meal with other people. Each could take it in turns to host the meal. You could get into trying new recipes, or have different themes for each occasion. You might also enjoy cooking for others - some cakes for a neighbour, perhaps. Again, this highlights the social aspect of diet, something that should not be neglected.

If cooking is not your thing, treat yourself every now and then. It does not have to be an expensive meal in a restaurant, some fish and chips from the local shop can be just as nice!

There are numerous food supplements available these days, from vitamins to zinc, fish oils and so on. You may find some of these useful - I personally take magnesium, kelp and a couple of other supplements at the moment. Do your research, speak to your doctor and, as with exercise, don't get drawn in to the latest fad.

As well as taking supplements, we should also consider medication. This can

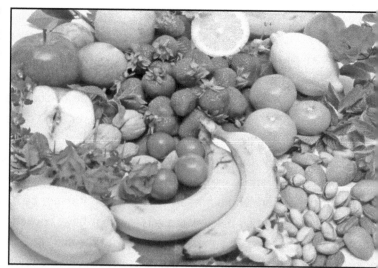

be a difficult area as GPs vary considerable in their outlook. I am lucky in that my local GP is not one to prescribe drugs for every little thing. In contrast, I remember my grandmother at one time being on around 15 pills a day - and half of those were to counter the side effects of the others! Again, do your research, see if there are other methods that will help with particular ailments. Be sure only to deal with accredited practitioners in their field.

Alongside food, comes alcohol. We are all aware of the dangers of of excess drinking - particularly as we age and balance becomes more of an issue. However, there is often a strong social aspect to drinking and, in moderation, drinks like wine may even be good for us!

If isolated, it can be easy to fall into the trap of heavy drinking. It becomes a form of self-medication, but is a slippery slope to potentially severe health issues. So

monitor your intake, ration yourself necessary. Whether it is food or booze, the simplest method of abstention is not to have it in the house. I know that if I buy a packet of nice shortbread biscuits, they can disappear in one sitting. That's okay now and then, but every day? So, biscuits rarely make it into the shopping basket.

Another aspect of food is to grow your own. If you are lucky enough to have a garden, set aside some space. Or look at local allotments and gardening clubs. Not only will you get free food, you will also meet new people.

A major Systema health practice is fasting - taking a break from food and drink for a specificed period of time. If you wish to try this, again proceed and slowly and follow medical advice. Fasting is an ancient practice, used in religious and health traditions around the world for thousands of years. All animals do it occasionally, either by choice or by circumstance.

Thousands of studies have found fasting to have positive effects on obesity, cardiovascular disease, autoimmune disorders, diabetes, skin disease, gastrointestinal disease, arthritis and more. On a physical level, it is very good for the internal system to get a break. This gives the body a chance to remove toxins and eliminate weak and dying cells. On a psychological level, fasting helps strengthen self-control and can assist in weaning ourselves off of unhealthy foods or to start a new diet. There are three forms of fasting:

Dry Fasting - abstaining from all food and liquid.

Juice Fasting - abstaining from food and drink except water and pure vegetable and fruit juices.

Modified Fasting - eating only small amounts of food, usually raw fruit, and steamed veg, or drinking herbal teas or broths.

The best way to start is with a short fasting period, say the 16/8 method. This means that we restrict all eating to a 16 hour period in the day, then fast for eight. Most of us do this anyway, unless you get up at night to snack! From here, you can gradually extend the fasting period. At first, allow yourself a little water or herbal tea.

When ready, you can try a full 24 hour fast of whichever type suits you best. If you find that too hard, then try removing an ingredient out of your diet, for example meat or dairy products. Where practical you should try and retain your daily routine, depending on safety, of course. You can prepare for a fast by having a day of lighter eating to help your body adjust. Vegetarian meals are best, as animal products are harder to digest. So the day before you might try smaller meals of steamed veg, fruit and so on.

At the beginning of a fast you may experience hunger pains and slight headaches, but this should pass quickly. Your body may start ejecting toxins leading to a unpleasant taste in the mouth. Simply

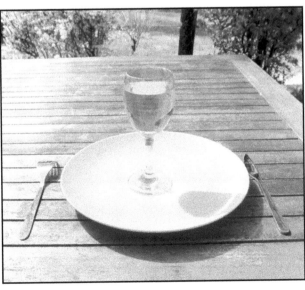

rinse your mouth with warm water. When you fast, nonessential tissues, like fat, are used for fuel. During the initial period of conservation, the body functions with the same degree of efficiency and blood sugar levels remain fairly constant. After 24 hours, the body's metabolism can slow by as much as 75%, so for longer fasts be sure to include plenty of rest.

Once your fast is over, ease back into solid foods. Start with light meals, do not binge as this will place a heavy demand on your body and be counter productive. Lastly, take the fasting process as an opportunity to review your overall diet and eating habits. Note, perhaps, how eating patterns are attached to certain emotional states and do your best to maintain a full, well balanced diet.

So, to recap, start with a short fast and work up to 24 hours. Always check with your doctor prior to fasting, especially if you have an existing medical condition, are on prescription drugs and so on. Be aware of your activities during fasting and do nothing that may be dangerous if you become light headed.

HOBBIES

Let's now consider social issues, feelings of isolation and so on. If we are reasonably mobile, there are usually a huge range of local clubs for all sorts of activities - from model railways to crafting to alpine walking. Check in your area to see what is available.

Likewise, there are often evening classes or courses available for learning new languages, a musical instrument, art appreciation and so on. It's never to late to learn something new, and exercising the mind is just as important as exercising the body.

What if we are not mobile though, or, as at time of writing, in some kind of lockdown?

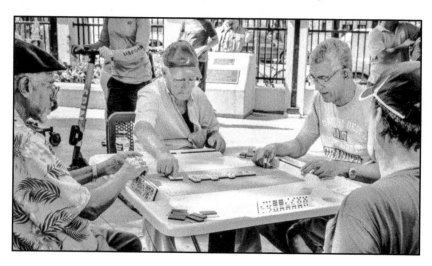

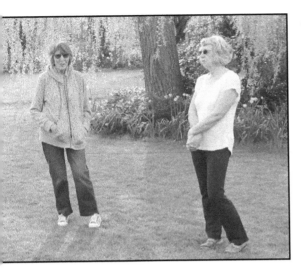

elderly neighbours, it is nice to check on them now and then. A ten minute chat over a cup of tea can go a long way to overcoming feelings of isolation.

OUTLOOK

Stress is inevitable but, as the saying goes, suffering is optional. If I had to distil stress management down into one phrase it would be this:

ook into keeping in contact with people ia the range of social media available. Aside from conventional texts and phone calls, there are various video apps available, not just for two but for whole groups of people.

Can you do something to change or improve the current situation? Then do it. If not, then stop worrying about it.

Why not organise regular chats with groups of friends? I realise that new technology may appear daunting if you have never used it, but local libraries and the like often run "how to" courses in computers. If not, perhaps a family member or neighbour can help get you started.

Easy to say, of course, not always so easy to do. But I you find yourself worried about things, try making a list of them. Then divide into "can change" or "can't change." Then take the first column and write down possible courses of action to take.

Another possibility via the internet are on-line courses, again a chance to learn a new skill and hopefully meet new people.

For example, you might have noisy neighbours. Possible actions include talking

On the flip side, if you are a younger person and have

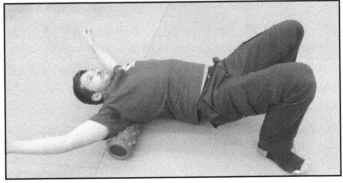

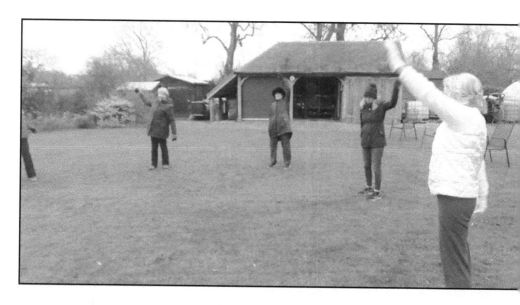

to them (perhaps they don't realise they are being a nuisance), buying earplugs, complaining to the relevant authorities, and so on.

For the things we cannot change - perhaps a chronic medical condition - we have to learn acceptance and then explore methods of managing its effects. The same applies to situations such as bereavement and other major life events. Again, I refer you to *Don't Worry* for detailed advice on these issues.

Outside of that, try to keep a positive mental attitude. There is a saying that what goes into the body is nourishment, what comes out is waste. That applies mentally as well as physically. Exposing ourselves to constant negativity will have an impact on our well-being.

Learn to put things into perspective and look for the silver lining in every situation. If you can, get out into nature every now and then I always find that a tonic. Social media while useful, can be a bad influence in some ways - you never have to look far for an argument on-line. So monitor your use - if you find yourself laying awake at night thinking about the message you are going to post tomorrow, then perhaps ease back on your on-line activities!

To encourage positivity, keeping an active and enquiring mind. Keep yourself up to date on current events, read, listen to new music, write your own! Again, if these things are difficult, then think back to your childhood times, or a time in your life when you were happy, draw strength from that. We have mention several times the notion of being "child-like" in our movement, so explore the concept of play in what you do -

whether that be through movement and dance, or playing board-games, or chess, for example.

In short, don't be worried about trying new things, change your routine every now and then, buy some new clothes, maybe visit a place you have never been to. If you can't get out, watch some documentaries or travel programs, get as much inter-action as you can with the outside world.

CONCLUSIONS

I hope you have enjoyed this book and find some useful things in it. Whether you use it to get a foundation before joining a class or are practicing solo at home, take your time to work through - there is a lot of material here, months, at least! Always train with an eye to the Four Pillars and you won't go far wrong.

And I emphasise again, think of your work as activity rather than exercise. Incorporate everything into your regular movements, into your daily life, into all that you do, that is when the true benefits arise.

If you do have any questions or comments, please feel free to get in touch with me, contact details are at the back of the book. Please also feel free to share your experiences, either direct, or via our Facebook page. Keep a positive outlook, stay mentally young and fresh, breathe, move and flow!

Good Health and Happy Training!

RESOURCES

Mikhail Ryabko
Systema HQ Moscow   www.systemaryabko.com

Vladimir Vasiliev
Systema HQ Toronto   www.russianmartialart.com

Cutting Edge Systema   www.systemauk.com
      www.facebook.com/groups/CuttingEdgeSystema
E-mail systemauk@outlook.com
Books & Instructional films   www.systemafilms.com

RECOMMENDED READING

Strikes - Vladimir Vasiliev & Scott Meredith

Let Every Breath - Vladimir Vasiliev

Secrets of the Russian Blade Masters - Vladimir Vasiliev

The Systema Manual - Major Konstantin Komarov

Other books by Robert Poyton

Systema Solo Training
Systema Partner Training
Systema Awareness Training
Systema Voices
Fitness Over 40
Don't Worry - A Guide to Stress Management
The Eight Brocades Qigong Exercise

Lightning Source UK Ltd.
Milton Keynes UK
UKHW051122231121
394456UK00008B/768

9 781637 526